W0111315

Microbiological
Hazards
of Infusion Therapy

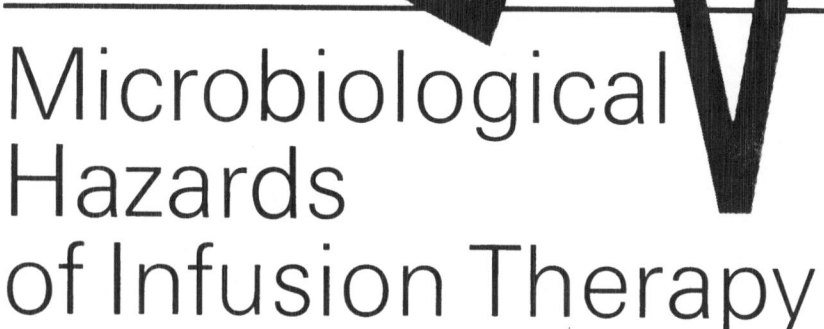

Microbiological
Hazards
of Infusion Therapy

Edited by
I. Phillips
P. D. Meers
P. F. D'Arcy

Proceedings of an International
Symposium held at the University
of Sussex, England, March 1976

MTP

Published by

MTP Press Ltd
St Leonard's House
St Leonardgate
Lancaster, Lancs
England

Copyright © 1976 MTP Press Ltd
Softcover reprint of the hardcover 1st edition 1976

*No part of this book may be reproduced
in any form without permission from
the publishers except for the quotation
of brief passages for review purposes.*

ISBN-13: 978-94-011-6181-7   e-ISBN-13: 978-94-011-6179-4
DOI: 10.1007/ 978-94-011-6179-4

Typeset in Great Britain by Lancashire Typesetting Co Ltd, Bolton

Contents

List of Contributors

Dr M. C. ALLWOOD
Department of Pharmacy, University of Manchester, Manchester M13 9PL

Professor P. F. D'ARCY
The Queen's University of Belfast, Lisburn Road, Belfast BT9 7BL, Northern Ireland

Dr R. E. DIXON
Bacterial Diseases Division, Bureau of Epidemiology, Center for Disease Control, Public Health Service, US Department of Health, Education and Welfare, Atlanta, Georgia 30333, USA

Dr A. M. GEDDES
Department of Communicable and Tropical Disease, East Birmingham Hospital, Birmingham B9 5ST

Dr R. HAMBLETON
Department of Pharmacy, University of Manchester, Manchester M13 9PL

Dr B. S. JENKINS
Department of Medicine, St Thomas's Hospital Medical School, London SE1 7EH

Dr D. G. MAKI
Infectious Disease Unit, University of Wisconsin Hospitals, 484 Medical Sciences Building, 1300 University Avenue, Madison, Wisconsin 53706, USA

Dr P. D. MEERS
Public Health Laboratory, Greenbank Hospital, Plymouth PL4 8NN, Devon

Professor I. PHILLIPS
Department of Microbiology, St Thomas's Hospital Medical School, London SE1 7EH

Professor Sir Robert WILLIAMS
Director, Public Health Laboratory Service, Colindale, London NW9 5EQ

Preface

All too often the fruits of modern medicine are blighted by avoidable infection when patients on whom technical skills have been lavished die or lose a benefit they might otherwise have enjoyed. Although such a loss is expensive both in terms of human tragedy and of wasted time and resources, scant attention is paid to its prevention compared with that which goes into the development and use of the advanced techniques which so often bring infections in their train. The intravascular route for biochemical, pharmacological, nutritional and other physiological support and monitoring necessary to patients undergoing many of the demanding modern medical procedures opens a channel through which infection all too easily finds a way. When it does it may be unsuspected and undetected until too late by those whose attention is fixed on the end they seek while forgetting that the means they use can produce preventable disease.

The largest medical use of the intravascular route is for 'intravenous therapy'. Lip-service is paid to the idea that this carries a significant morbidity and mortality, but surprisingly little has been done to measure its incidence or design measures to avoid it. In the early 1970s, the medical and pharmaceutical professions, and the lay public, were startled by the realization of the microbiological threat to patients infused with products which had been subject to manufacturing error in their design or production. Paradoxically, this may have diverted attention from the incomparably more common problem of the infections that are introduced during the bedside phase of the use of initially sterile solutions and delivery apparatus.

The Symposium, of which these are the proceedings, was planned to draw together as much information as possible on the microbiological dangers to patients which may arise during the manufacture and use of intravenous fluids, together with relevant data on their packaging and delivery, and on the different clinical syndromes which result when precautions fail and infection follows. It is hoped that it will serve to put the subject into proper perspective and to highlight the problems and in particular to redress the imbalance that exists in many people's minds between the importance of intrinsic (manufacturing) and extrinsic (in-use) contamination, so that the latter will attract the attention it deserves and urgently needs for its correction.

Travenol Laboratories Limited sponsored the Symposium and provided the administrative services needed to run it. The contributors and editors are deeply grateful for the opportunity that this has given them to reach a wider public with a message whose importance daily grows greater. The editors acknowledge the helpful collaboration of our publisher, and the skill of Mrs Judy Fagelston who transcribed the discussions.

Opening address
Sir Robert Williams

The most dramatic example of the triumphs of intravenous therapy must be in the treatment of cholera; a disease that had a mortality of up to 20% now reduced to $0 \cdot 2\%$ or less, simply by intravenous saline, often given in vast quantities and without any necessary contribution from antibiotics.

In most parts of the world intravenous therapy on the cholera scale is virtually unknown, but the number of hospital patients who have need for some intravenous fluid replacement is very large indeed and like all treatments it has its hazards—the topic for this symposium arranged by Travenol Laboratories, which it gives me great pleasure to open.

Prolonged intravenous therapy was recognized many years ago as carrying a risk of staphylococcal septicaemia, and indeed for a time constituted a major aetiological source of such disease. This led to much investigation on the importance of particular forms of intravenous catheters, study of drip-site hygiene and so forth. Like most hazards it is best avoided by avoidance of the cause: prolonged infusion at one site.

The hazards of infusion with high nutrient fluids have also been recognized for a good many years, with demonstration of the risk of growth in the fluid, especially of *Candida* and other fungi.

The risks of bacteraemia arising from non-nutrient infusion fluids has been recognized more recently, highlighted by a small number of outbreaks which arose from contamination at place of manufacture with bacteria that are ordinarily very rarely found responsible even for a single case of bacteraemia, let alone for an epidemic. Bacteraemia attributable to Gram-negative bacilli has been a topic of increasing interest in any case in recent years and in consequence there has been increasing attention to identification of the bacteria isolated, and recognition that, given the right opportunities, i.e. dose, susceptible patient and so forth, many of the bacteria classically regarded as non-pathogenic can produce fatal disease.

During the symposium you will undoubtedly be hearing much of the problems of recognizing incipient outbreaks of infection arising from contaminated fluids, and of the problems of preventing the contamination. These are indeed matters of concern to all who work in hospitals—in the wards or in the laboratory—and I am sure that the ensuing discussions will be of great value.

SECTION ONE

Sources of Contamination
Chairman:
Professor I. Phillips

1

Containers and closures
R. Hambleton and M. C. Allwood

1.1 INTRODUCTION

An essential aspect of the production of sterile fluids for hospital use is the container–closure system in which such products are packaged. The container–closure system is the means whereby the fluid, once sterilized, is protected from contamination until the time when it is used. Containers must therefore comply with several requirements if they are to be suitable for sterile fluids. These requirements may be summarized as follows:

(a) They must be chemically compatible with the fluid.
(b) They must be able to withstand the method of sterilization.
(c) They must be able to maintain the sterility of the fluid from the moment when the sterilization process has been completed.
(d) They must permit the safe withdrawal of the contents for use.

These rules inevitably embrace not only the container but also the closure and it is perhaps more correct to use the term container to include both the main body of the container and its closure. The importance of adequate container design is self evident when one considers that containers are subject to approval in the licensing of a product under the Medicines Act regulations.

1.2 MATERIALS USED FOR STERILE FLUID CONTAINERS

Sterile fluid containers are made of a variety of materials. Historically glass containers have been most commonly used but there is an increasing tendency for containers manufactured from plastics to be used.

1.2.1 Glass containers

Glass containers for sterile fluids may be made of soft (soda) glass, neutral or borosilicate glass. The European Pharmacopoeia[1] specifies three types of glass for parenteral injections. Glass type I is defined as 'glass commonly known as neutral glass having a high hydrolytic resistance due to the chemical composition of the glass itself'. This type is represented by borosilicate glass or by neutral glass containing barium compounds. Glass type II is defined as 'glass having a high hydrolytic resistance resulting from the appropriate treatment of the surface'. This is a sulphated soda glass. Glass type III, 'glass having only moderate hydrolytic resistance', is again a soft glass and is not intended for preparations in an aqueous vehicle. Thus for large volume parenteral injections the recommended materials are glass types I and II. Containers made of glass type II are not intended for re-use. In the United Kingdom most glass infusion containers are manufactured from soft glass although other European countries use both type I and type II containers.

Glass containers are heat-resistant and thus able to withstand the conditions of autoclaving though breakage of soft glass bottles may occur due to thermal shock during sterilization[2]. They are re-usable to an extent dependent on the type of glass and are generally inert, although untreated soda glass is readily attacked by alkaline solutions (e.g. sodium bicarbonate solutions) and even by sodium chloride and citrate solutions. Hair line cracks may develop in glass containers as a result of rough handling because of the fragile nature of the material. These may be responsible for the introduction of contaminating micro-organisms such as moulds[3]. The clarity of glass allows easy examination of the contents for particulate matter.

Glass bottles are considerably heavier than plastic containers of equivalent volume. A 500 ml MRC bottle of water may weigh over 1 kg whereas a filled plastic container of equivalent capacity may weigh only about half as much. This factor is important in respect of the handling and transportation of fluids in large numbers since it may contribute to accidental damage of the containers.

When glass containers are used for administering infusions they must be provided with airways inserted through the closures to permit the free flow of fluid through the giving set.

A serious disadvantage with glass containers is that they must be sealed by closures of a different material or materials. This is usually achieved by means of natural or synthetic rubber seals secured by aluminium screw caps or crimp-on rings. The use of such dissimilar materials as glass and rubber at the sealing surface may lead to potential hazards during autoclaving when the closures are under considerable stress. These stresses will be dealt with in more detail later but the effects of stress will be compounded by poorly fitting seals and by the different rates of expansion of the glass and aluminium screw caps[3,4].

All glass bottles must be inspected for damage and irregularity in manufacture, and must be washed free of particulate matter before use. Such activities are labour-intensive and thus expensive. Washing may itself introduce problems especially if the detergent used adheres firmly to the glass. Copious rinsing with filtered water is necessary after washing in order to ensure that all detergent and particulate matter is removed from the bottle. The problems of washing and inspection are multiplied if bottles are re-used. Re-use increases the likelihood of minor damage to containers (for instance chipping of the neck or lip). Such damage may be difficult to detect but can contribute to the failure of the seal during sterilization in an autoclave.

1.2.1.1 *Particulate contamination in glass containers*

It is generally accepted that fluids in glass containers are liable to contamination by foreign particulate matter. This occurs despite efforts to ensure that the fluid being packed is introduced in a particle-free condition. Fluids in soft glass containers may contain flakes of glass and this problem increases if such containers are re-used. The other main source of particulate contamination may be the rubber closure. Fragments of rubber may be detached from the closure during autoclaving and it has been claimed that some of the insoluble ingredients of rubber such as carbon black, zinc oxide, chalk and clay have been released into fluids. It has even been suggested that mould spores might be released into the fluid by the bursting of blisters in the closure[5-7]. Lacquers have been used in an attempt to prevent rubber closures shedding particles but since the lacquer is less flexible than rubber it may itself flake off when the rubber closures are flexed when introduced to the bottle neck. Particulate contamination from rubber closures has been reduced by means of teflon liners to rubber closures[8].

1.2.1.2 *Stresses on containers and closures during sterilization*

Glass bottles contain an air–liquid system in which the proportion of liquid to air varies according to the design of the bottle and whether or not the bottles are filled under a partial vacuum. During autoclaving the pressures generated within a container may be quite high because of the increase in air temperature and the expression of the liquid into the bottle head space. The ultimate pressure generated at sterilizing temperature is thus the sum of the partial pressures of both air and steam in the closed system and may be deduced from the equation[9].

$$P_2 = \frac{P_1 V_1 T_2 + P_1 + P_3}{T_1(V_1 - v)}$$

where P_2 = bottle pressure at sterilizing temperature (T_2)

P_1 = initial bottle pressure
P_3 = pressure of steam at T_2
T_1 = initial temperature (K)
T_2 = sterilizing temperature (K)
V_1 = initial head space volume
v = volume expansion of the fluid contents between T_1 and T_2.

Additional corrections might be made to account for the expansion of the glass and for volume differences introduced with different types of closure but these are extremely small and may be ignored for practical purposes.

Applying this equation to bottles shows that the absolute internal pressure may be greatly in excess of the pressure in the sterilizer chamber. The extent of this pressure differential is increased sharply when the volume of fluid exceeds about 80% of the total internal bottle capacity. The stress on the bottle closure is twofold. First the increase in temperature during autoclaving causes differential expansion of the metal cap and the glass bottle neck. As a result caps do not secure the rubber seals as tightly and screw caps may even back off (unscrew) a little under the influence of the reverse torque generated in the rubber closure when the caps were first screwed on. Second, the high pressure within the bottle forces the rubber seal upwards like a piston so that the aluminium caps may take on a distinct dome shape[3]. Thus, bottle closures which may have been adequate before sterilization may be stressed to the limit during sterilization.

Air may escape from a proportion of bottles when the closures are a poor fit on the bottle necks and on cooling such bottles develop a partial internal vacuum. Bottles in this state can take up contamination more readily than those without an internal vacuum.

1.2.1.3 Contamination hazards with bottles

Several instances have been reported where bottle contamination was thought to be caused by the introduction of contaminated spray-cooling water in the autoclave chamber[10–13]. When bottles are spray-cooled the pressure in the bottles is reduced and, if leakage of air has occurred, the bottle pressure will eventually be lower than in the autoclave chamber particularly if the sterilizer employs an air ballast to protect the bottles from pressure shock during spray-cooling. The internal vacuum may draw in spray-cooling water, and with it any contaminating organisms. An additional contamination risk is introduced in the area of the seal even if the bottles have not developed a vacuum because spray-cooling water will readily penetrate under aluminium caps and contaminate the bottle neck and the upper surface of the closure through which the giving set must eventually be introduced. The extent to which spray-cooling water penetrates beneath metal screw caps may depend upon the design of the autoclave. It has been reported that penetration was greater in those autoclaves employing an air ballast during spray-cooling than in those where no air ballast was employed[14].

The presence of contaminating organisms in the area of the bottle seal may bring about contamination during rough handling and when giving sets are introduced[3]. Recent work in our laboratory has shown that the ease with which organisms on the outside of rubber closures are introduced into bottles by the insertion of a giving set may ultimately depend on the design of the closure. The standard MRC relieved closure is much more difficult to swab clean than a similar closure with a shallow more accessible indentation at the giving set entry point. Many giving sets have a very wide bore 'needle' for insertion through the bottle cap. These are often difficult to push through the rubber and the distortion of the rubber may facilitate the entry of contaminating microorganisms. Should the bottle have an internal vacuum, the airway needle should be inserted before the giving set needle so that no unfiltered air can enter the bottle.

1.3 PLASTIC CONTAINERS

All types of plastic containers are, as previously discussed, lighter in weight than equivalent glass bottles. They are also more resistant to breakage during handling and transport. Since they are all single-use containers the problems of decontamination and washing associated with recycling do not arise. In fact, it is possible to manufacture such containers in a particle-free environment thus removing the need for any form of pretreatment prior to filling. Since the filling port is relatively small the chances of contamination occurring during this stage of manufacture are greatly reduced compared with glass bottles. Plastic containers are sealed by either heat or high (radio) frequency welding thus enabling a complete seal to be made without the use of rubber closures. The filling and sealing process can be carried out with one machine thus providing the possibility of a highly automatic process which reduces the chance of contamination from operators to a negligible level. There are machines available that blow mould, fill and seal plastic infusion packs in a continuous operation[15].

The sterilization of fluids in plastic packs poses additional problems for the pharmacist since the container must be protected during the autoclave cycle to prevent deformation and bursting[16]. Thus the pressure during the sterilization cycle must be the same in the autoclave chamber as in the infusion container. The usual method is to provide a steam–air mixture as the sterilization medium. Therefore, the design of this sterilization cycle is different from that employed for glass bottles and only recently have autoclaves been readily available for this purpose. Although the vapour pressure of steam inside the bag and in the autoclave chamber will be equal under sterilizing conditions, pressures inside the bag are increased principally by the expansion of the fluid and of any residual air trapped in the container. This must be balanced by the addition of air to the autoclave chamber. For such a situation, the atmosphere inside the chamber may no longer be homogenous, due to layering of the lighter steam above the heavier air. In order to maintain homogeneity, great care is required to create a turbulent system by provision of a fan inside the autoclave chamber, or by the continuous injection of a steam–air mixture into the bottom of the chamber.

A very important advantage offered by plastic packs over glass bottles is that, since they are presented as a completely enclosed sealed system, there is no possibility of contamination of the contents by spray-cooling water. Further, it may be possible to enclose the pack in an overwrap before sterilization, thus ensuring a completely sterile container for use.

At the present time two types of plastic are used widely for intravenous infusion packs; these are polyvinylchloride (PVC) and polyethylene.

1.3.1 Polyvinylchloride

PVC suitable for use in this field is composed of pure PVC polymer to which are added plasticizers and fillers thus producing a flexible and transparent film. The bags are manufactured by the sealing together of two separate sheets or from lay-flat tubing, by high-frequency welding. Due to the adaptability of the process, it is a relatively simple operation to seal into the bag the ports for the infusion set and additives. Such parts are readily protected from environmental contamination by tear-off over-seals, thus ensuring a sterile surface for set application until immediately before use. Labelling can be done before filling by simple printing techniques. Consequently, the filled bag can be placed in an overwrap prior to sterilization. In any case, it is essential to protect the contents of PVC bags by a moisture-impermeable outer container because of the high water permeability of PVC film. Under normal storage conditions up to 2% water loss per month can occur from the fluid in the unprotected bag[17]. It is therefore important that the bag is not removed from the outer-wrap until just before use (48 hours is the recommended maximum interval), otherwise the fluid composition will alter significantly.

Provided that all seals are efficiently made, the container is very resistant to rough handling. If the administration set port is suitably designed, needle insertion can be conducted with the minimum risk of touch contamination by the user. The principal concern with the use of PVC arises from the possibility of extractives being leached from the plastic into the fluid. Plasticizers, usually consisting of phthallate salts, are used to soften the polymer. Studies have shown that potentially toxic chemicals can be found in fluids packed in PVC bags[18]. Recent evidence has shown that negligible amounts of phthallate salts are leached into most infusions in PVC containers although there does appear to be significantly greater leaching into bags containing human blood[19]. Pharmacopoeial standards now include limits for extractives from containers used for blood products and aqueous fluids. It is clear that soluble extractives leach from PVC film due to an incomplete interaction between PVC and plasticizer during manufacture of the film. This risk can be reduced by the use of high quality material. Pin-holing of the film can also arise due to poor standards of manufacture. Such containers would usually be identified after sterilization due to the leakage of fluid.

Immediately prior to administration it is recommended practice to examine the fluid for particulate contamination and cloudiness due to bacterial growth. Since PVC film is clear when not hydrated, any cloudiness can readily be detected although printing may obscure areas of the container. A problem which occurs during administration is the inability of nurses to assess the volume of fluid remaining in the container at any particular time, but an important advantage compared with glass bottles is the absence of an airway, since the bag is completely collapsible. This also reduces the risk of air embolism. At least one survey has indicated that the nursing staff prefer intravenous fluids presented in plastic packs[19].

A final point related to PVC bags concerns the common practice of adding drugs to infusions. It has been suggested that some drugs are liable to sorbtion into the plastic[20].

1.3.2 Polythene

Polythene provides a suitable material for the fabrication of fluid containers. Relatively high-density polyethylene must be employed which has a sufficiently high melting temperature. Unfortunately, this leads to some loss of pliability and an increase in the opacity of containers. The containers are readily made by a blow-moulding process to produce a sealed unit. It is, therefore, possible to produce a particle-free container which can be unsealed immediately before filling. The major technological difficulty of using polythene for infusion containers is that the material does not lend itself to the provision of secondary ports or to welding of overwraps to protect the giving set port. Consequently ports, though sealed, may be unprotected from environmental or personnel contamination before use. Since it is not possible to print on the surface of polythene, labelling must be carried out after sterilization, so that the bag cannot be overwrapped before autoclaving. It is, therefore, not possible to present a sterile port for giving set needle insertion. The seal is either cut off with sterile scissors or a tear-off system is adopted. During sterilization, the container must be placed in a rigid holder to prevent permanent physical deformation of the plastic; this may reduce the rate of heat transfer and therefore prolong the sterilization cycle.

Since polythene is impermeable to water vapour, loss of moisture does not occur during storage and a moisture-impermeable overwrap is unnecessary. Unfortunately, polythene is somewhat opaque dependent on the density of polymer, and examination for particles and cloudiness is difficult. Since the pack possesses some degree of rigidity it may not collapse completely during infusion of the contents and therefore the drip-rate may fall as the withdrawal of liquid proceeds. This may encourage the addition of an airway (of some sort or other) to maintain the fluid flow. Since there is no additive port, drugs must be introduced directly through the wall of the bag thus introducing a potential passage for microbial entry into the pack.

Since pure polythene can be used, the possibility of soluble extractives being present in the fluid is negligible, and the sorbtion of drug additives appears to be far less significant into polythene compared with PVC film.

One area in which polythene has a definite advantage is in the production of alkaline infusions such as high concentration sodium bicarbonate solutions. PVC is permeable to carbon dioxide and this can lead to a deterioration in sodium bicarbonate infusions during storage. In contrast, polythene is completely impermeable to carbon dioxide.

Sterile infusion fluid containers made both of glass and plastics will no doubt continue to be used during the forseeable future. The glass containers may be especially useful in satisfying the demand for special infusions in particular hospitals but there is an increasing tendency toward the use of plastic packs for the more commonly used infusions. It is relatively simple to prepare sterile fluids in collapsible plastic bags. The major advantage is that the likelihood of microbial contamination of the fluid is greatly reduced during sterilization, storage and use. The absence of an airway offers another safeguard against contamination during infusion. The major problems related to toxic extractives from PVC film can largely be overcome by the use of the highest quality material. It is not therefore surprising that infusion fluids packed in plastic packs are becoming increasingly popular with both pharmacists and clinical staff.

In conclusion, one may say that the microbial safety of intravenous infusions depends to an extent upon the containers in which they are prepared and presented for use. With this in mind, considerable care should be taken with the design of containers and closures in an endeavour to minimize contamination risks from these sources.

References

1. European Pharmacopoeia. (1971). **2**, Glass containers for injectable preparations, p. 65. (Council of Europe)
2. Lomax, J. (1972). Fracture analysis as an aid to quality control. *Glass*, March, 2
3. Myers, J. A. (1974). Microbial contamination of packaged fluids after sterilization. *Pharm. J.*, **212**, 308
4. Beverley, S., Hambleton, R. and Allwood, M. C. (1974). Leakage of spray cooling water into topical water bottles. *Pharm. J.*, **212**, 306
5. Garvan, J. M. and Gunner, B. W. (1963). Intravenous fluids: 'A solution containing such particles must not be used'. *Med. J. Australia*, **2**, 140
6. Garvan, J. M. and Gunner, B. W. (1964). The harmful effects of particles in intravenous fluids. *Med. J. Australia*, **2**, 1
7. Garvan, J. M. and Gunner, B. W. (1971). Particulate contamination of intravenous fluids. *Br. J. Clin. Pract.*, **25**, 119
8. Ernerot, L., Helmstein, I. and Sandel, E. (1970). Some factors influencing the measured content of particulate matter in infusion fluids. *Acta Pharm. Suecica*, **1**, 501
9. Allwood, M. C., Hambleton, R. and Beverley, S. (1975). Pressure changes in bottles during sterilization by autoclaving. *J. Pharm. Sci.*, **64**, 333
10. Phillips, I., Eykyn, S. and Laker, M. (1972). Outbreak of hospital infection caused by contaminated autoclaved fluids. *Lancet*, **i**, 1258
11. Joynson, D. H. M., Howells, C. H. C., Liddington, R. and Williams, A. (1975). Contamination of fluids from a hospital pharmacy. *J. Hyg., Camb.*, **75**, 87
12. Spatz, M., Ho, N. F. H., Curtiss, E. G. and Patel, J. A. (1973). The sterility of a screw capped bottle system containing irrigating solutions. *Drug Intell. Clin. Pharm.*, **7**, 463
13. Lapage, S. P., Johnson, R. and Holmes, B. (1973). Bacteria from intravenous fluids. *Lancet*, **ii**, 284
14. Beverley, S., Hambleton, R. and Allwood, M. C. (1973). Bottle leakage and autoclave design. *Pharm. J.*, **211**, 321
15. Groves, M. (1973). *Parenteral Products*, p. 146 (London: Heinemann)
16. Schuck, L. J. (1973). Steam sterilization of solutions in plastic bottles. Presented at the *International Symposium on Sterilization and Sterility testing of Biological Substances*, Madrid
17. Macdonald, A. (1974). Permeation of Water Vapour through plastic containers for intravenous infusion fluids. *J. Hosp. Pharm.*, September, 70
18. Jaeger, R. J. and Rubin R. J. (1972). Migration of Phthallate Ester Plasticiser from Polyvinyl Chloride Blood Bags into stored Human Blood and its Localisation in Human Tissues. *N. Engl. J. Med.*, **287**, 1114
19. Williams, A. and James, B. (1973). An evaluation of the Degree of Acceptance of Intravenous Fluids in Plastic Packs. *J. Hosp. Pharm.*, June, 130
20. Moorhatch, P. and Chiou, W. L. (1974). Interactions between drugs and plastic intravenous fluid bags. Part i: Sorption studies on 17 drugs. *Am. J. Hosp. Pharm.*, **31**, 72

2

Growth properties of microorganisms in infusion fluid and methods of detection
D. G. Maki

2.1 GROWTH PROPERTIES OF MICROORGANISMS IN FLUIDS FOR INFUSION

2.1.1 Historical basis

Infusion therapy has been employed worldwide for over 45 years, yet ironically the hazard of iatrogenic septicaemic infection only gradually became recognized in the late 1950s[1].

A myriad of studies appeared over the next decade but dealt almost exclusively with events occurring at the most distal portion of the infusion system, phlebitis and septicaemia related to indwelling plastic catheters. In 1953, Michaels and Ruebner from Great Britain published a startling and now historic report implicating microbial contamination of infusion fluid in the genesis of two cases of Gram-negative septicaemia[2]; the pathogens exhibited differential growth abilities in two parenteral solutions. Yet, the rest of the infusion apparatus and particularly infusion fluid remained widely unappreciated as a source of contamination until 1970. Between July 1970 and March 1971, many hospitals in the United States experienced epidemics of nosocomial septicaemia with *Enterobacter cloacae* and *Erwinia* (*herbicola–lathyri* group; proposed designation *Enterobacter agglomerans*[3]) caused by *intrinsic* contamination of one manufacturer's infusion products[1,4-8].

During our early epidemic, investigations at the United States Center for Disease Control (USCDC) before identification of the source of Abbott's contamination as intrinsic (during manufacture), surveys of infusion systems manufactured by Abbott, Baxter and Cutter Laboratories sampled during clinical use in the hospital had shown 6·8–35% rates of fluid contamination, with multiple organisms[4,8-10]. However, with rare exceptions only *Klebsiella*, *Enterobacter* and *Serratia* which comprise the tribe Klebsielleae were found in concentrations greater than 10 organisms per ml. Moreover, in the nationwide outbreak and in the three reports published up to that time of septicaemia caused by contaminated intravenous fluid[2,11,12] the major pathogens were members of the tribe Klebsielleae.

Then, as now, 5% dextrose in water (D5%/W) was virtually synonymous with intravenous therapy and along with other solutions containing glucose was by far the most frequently used parenteral solution in US hospitals. During the nationwide epidemic more than 90% of affected patients received glucose-containing fluids[8].

Enterobacter aerogenes can fix atmospheric nitrogen[13]. In addition, many members of the tribe Klebsielleae are facultative psychrophiles and grow well at room temperature[14]. Thus we postulated that microorganisms of this tribe possess a selective ability to proliferate in glucose-containing infusion fluids at room temperature and in January 1971 undertook a study to test this hypothesis[15].

2.1.2 *In vitro* studies

2.1.2.1 *Studies with conventional fluids at the USCDC*

(a) *Methods*—An *in vitro* study of microbial growth in infusion fluid was designed to simulate as closely as possible the microbial ecology attending contamination of conventional infusion fluid both during manufacture and during use in the hospital (Table 2.1). A total of 106 strains representing 9 genera and 13 species, including 51 strains of the tribe Klebsielleae, 5 strains of *Candida albicans* and 49 strains of other bacteria (*Escherichia coli*, *Pseudomonas aeruginosa*, *Proteus* spp., *Acinetobacter* and *Staphylococcus* spp.) were selected for study. Nearly all were clinical isolates from hospitals uninvolved in the national epidemic. Growth of all 106 strains was evaluated in Abbott's D5%/W, 18 strains from all 9 genera in normal (0·9%) saline, and 1 strain each of *E. cloacae* and *Esch. coli*

TABLE 2.1   Features of study design which enhance clinical applicability of *in vitro* studies of microbial growth in infusion fluid

---

1. Test wide variety of microbial species and representative number of strains, ideally all clinical isolates

2. Emphasis upon most heavily utilized products (i.e. 5% dextrose in water) and test in all major commercial brands

3. Exclusion of organic sources of nitrogen from test solutions (e.g. twice wash the inoculum)

4. Realistic inoculum size (e.g. approximately 1 organism/ml)

5. Incubation in original container at room temperature (25 °C) without continuous agitation or other manipulations that deviate from conventional clinical use of infusion fluid

6. Frequent sampling in the first 24 hours

---

in D5%/W manufactured by Abbott, Baxter, Cutter and McGaw. Test organisms were twice washed in sterile normal saline and an inoculum was introduced directly into freshly opened bottles of infusion fluid to give an initial (0-time) concentration of between 1 and 10 organisms per ml. Bottles were incubated without agitation at 25 °C and sampled in triplicate by conventional pour plate techniques, at 0-time and at 3, 6, 12, 24 and 48 hours. At each sampling, the bottle was carefully inspected under a bright lamp for turbidity, "Schlieren" or other visual evidence of microbial growth. The concentration at each sampling point for each strain was normalized to an initial concentration of 1 organism per ml.

(b) *Results*—This *in vitro* experiment conclusively demonstrated differential growth properties of representative nosocomial pathogens in infusion fluids which had been predicted on the basis of known biochemical properties and clinical and epidemiological observations. As seen in Figure 2.1, strains of Klebsielleae proliferated rapidly at 25 °C reaching logarithmic phase by 6–12 hours and attaining a mean normalized concentration for the group of $1 \cdot 1 \times 10^5$ per ml at 24 hours and $1 \cdot 7 \times 10^6$ per ml at 48 hours. *E. cloacae* and *E. agglomerans*, the major pathogens in the ongoing nationwide epidemic, were among the most rapid growers (Table 2.2). Only 1 of 51 strains of the Klebsielleae tribe tested, an *E. cloacae* strain, failed to grow. This was confirmed by repeat testing. In contrast, 48 of the 49 other strains failed to grow or more commonly died ($p < 0 \cdot 001$). One acinetobacter isolate repeatedly attained 24-hour concentrations of 10^3 to 10^4 organisms per ml. The five strains of *Candida albicans* grew only very slowly reaching a mean 24-hour concentration of 31 organisms per ml (Figure 2.1, Table 2.2).

TABLE 2.2   Growth of 105 strains in D5%/W at 25 °C*

Organism	No. strains tested	Mean (standard error) concentration at 24 h (organisms/ml)†
Tribe Klebsielleae		
E. cloacae	11	$2 \cdot 9 \ (0 \cdot 8) \times 10^5$
S. marcescens	10	$1 \cdot 3 \ (0 \cdot 5) \times 10^5$
E. agglomerans (Erwinia)	6	$1 \cdot 1 \ (0 \cdot 2) \times 10^5$
E. liquefaciens	3	$3 \cdot 8 \ (1 \cdot 1) \times 10^4$
Kl. pneumoniae	10	$3 \cdot 0 \ (2 \cdot 5) \times 10^4$
E. hafnia	5	$7 \cdot 0 \ (3 \cdot 4) \times 10^3$
E. aerogenes	6	$5 \cdot 2 \ (2 \cdot 5) \times 10^3$
Total	51	$1 \cdot 1 \ (0 \cdot 2) \times 10^5$
Non-tribe Klebsielleae		
Esch. coli	11	$0 \cdot 7 \ (0 \cdot 2)$
Acinetobacter (Herellea)	3‡	$0 \cdot 2 \ (0 \cdot 2)$
Ps. aeruginosa	10	$0 \cdot 1 \ (0 \cdot 1)$
Proteus species	12	$0 \cdot 1 \ (0 \cdot 1)$
Staphylococcus species	13	$0 \cdot 0$
Total	49	$3 \cdot 1 \ (2 \cdot 7)$
C. albicans	5	$31 \cdot 3 \ (4 \cdot 1)$

* Maki and Martin[15]
† Normalized to an initial zero-time concentration of $1 \cdot 0$ organism/ml
‡ Excludes one strain of Acinetobacter that grew well ($1 \cdot 3 \times 10^3$ organisms per ml at 24 hours)

Evidence of microbial growth visible to the unaided eye could not be detected at any time even at 48 hours when many strains of the tribe Klebsielleae had attained concentrations exceeding 10^6 per ml.

The tested strain of Esch. coli failed to grow in any of the four manufacturers' brands of D5%/W. However, the E. cloacae strain grew well in all four manufacturers' fluid (Table 2.2).

None of the 18 strains tested grew in normal saline in the first 24 hours of incubation; however, over 48 hours, three Klebsielleae strains multiplied one log (mean = 23 organisms per ml).

2.1.2.2 Other studies with conventional fluids

Other investigators have also studied microbial growth in conventional infusion fluids[2,5,16–20]. However, the clinical applicability of many of these studies has been compromised in part by relatively few species and

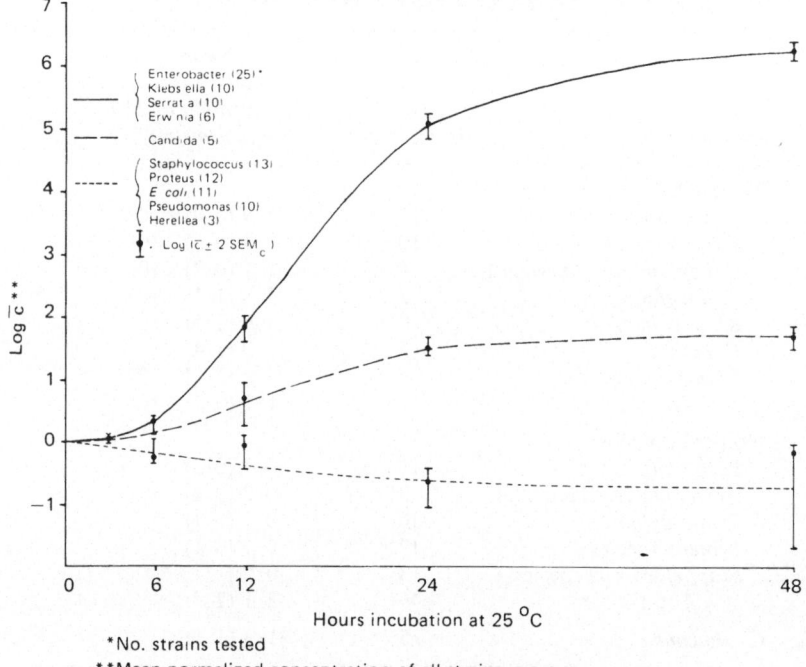

Figure 2.1 Growth curves of 106 microbial strains in D5%/W at 25 C. Numbers in parentheses indicate number of strains tested with equal mean normalized concentration of all strains in group. (From Maki and Martin[15], courtesy of *J. Infect. Dis.*)

strains tested[2,5,16-20], by failure to wash inocula[17,19,20], and particularly by large inoculum size, usually exceeding 10^4 organisms per ml[2,5,17-20]. Despite these limitations, results have been in relatively close agreement with the findings of our study which employed a large number of species and strains and stringently attempted to duplicate *in vivo* conditions (Table 2.1).

2.1.2.3 *Studies with fluids for total parenteral nutrition*

In the past 10 years intravenous administration of hypertonic glucose solutions with protein hydrolysates by total parenteral nutrition (TPN) has been shown to be a highly effective means of alimentation. However, in the first several years TPN began to be used widely,' from 1969–73, many hospitals reported extraordinary rates of associated septicaemia,

TABLE 2.3 Growth of fungi and bacteria in casein hydrolysate–50% dextrose total parenteral nutrition solution*

Organism	Organisms per ml†				
	0 (time)	12 (h)	24 (h)	48 (h)	7 (days)
C. albicans	1	24·0	$2·4 \times 10^3$	T	T
T. glabrata	1	15·0	$1·7 \times 10^3$	T	T
S. marcescens	1	28·0	$4·5 \times 10^3$	T	T
Kl. pneumoniae	1	12·0	$2·2 \times 10^3$	T	T
Staph. aureus	1	5·0	$1·4 \times 10^3$	T	T
Esch. coli	1	3·0	$1·1 \times 10^3$	$1·7 \times 10^6$	T
E. cloacae	1	4·7	96·0	$1·0 \times 10^6$	T
Pr. mirabilis	1	1·9	27·0	$7·2 \times 10^4$	T
Ps. aeruginosa	1	2·7	1·6	1·1	0·13

* Goldmann et al.[25]
† Mean concentration for five test strains of each organism, normalized to an inoculum of one organism per ml
T = Turbid

ranging as high as 23–27%. Inexplicably, *Candida* spp. were implicated in over half of these infections, many of which were fatal[21]. Early studies[22–24] indicated that *Candida* was able to multiply in TPN fluids, but whether this was a selective ability of *Candida* was less clear.

TABLE 2.4 Growth of fungi and bacteria in synthetic amino acid–50% dextrose total parenteral nutrition solution*

Organism	Organisms per ml†				
	0 (time)	12 (h)	24 (h)	48 (h)	7 (days)
C. albicans	1	8·5	49·0	$1·7 \times 10^2$	$1·7 \times 10^3$
T. glabrata	1	4·5	16·0	33·0	$6·5 \times 10^3$
S. marcescens	1	2·5	3·0	0·77	1·5
Kl. pneumoniae	1	0·63	0·15	0·06	0·05
Staph. aureus	1	0·66	0·24	0·01	0·09
Esch. coli	1	0·89	0·67	0·46	0·18
E. cloacae	1	0·62	0·16	0·06	0·06
Pr. mirabilis	1	0·67	0·52	0·23	0·12
Ps. aeruginosa	1	0·30	0·12	0·02	0·06

* Goldmann et al.[25]
† Mean concentration for five test strains of each organism, normalized to an inoculum of one organism per ml

In 1972, Goldmann, Martin and Worthington, at the Center for Disease Control, following an identical protocol extended our study of microbial growth in conventional infusion fluid to solutions for TPN[25]. Their results with 45 strains (Table 2.3, Figure 2.2) showed that *Candida albicans*, *Torulopsis glabrata*, *Serratia marcescens*, *Kl. pneumoniae* and *Staph. aureus* proliferate luxuriantly in a commercial TPN solution prepared from casein hydrolysate and 50% dextrose (mean 24-hour concentration, 10^3 per ml). Gross turbidity was apparent within 48 hours with most strains that grew. Among these organisms, however, only *Candida* and *Torulopsis* were able to grow, considerably more slowly (mean 48-hour concentration for *Candida* $1 \cdot 7 \times 10^2$ per ml), in a synthetic amino acid–50% dextrose

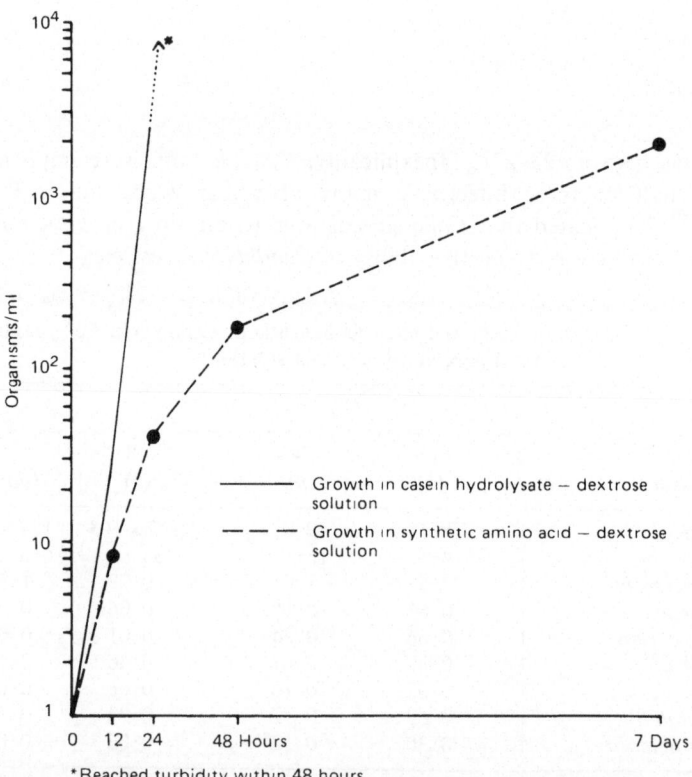

*Reached turbidity within 48 hours

Figure 2.2 Growth of five strains of *Candida albicans* in solutions for total parenteral nutrition. (From Goldmann *et al.*[25], courtesy of *Am. J. Surg.*)

solution (Table 2.4). None of the organisms grew in either solution when refrigerated at 4° C. With minor variations, Gelbart, *et al.*[18] and Sanderson and Deitel[26] have confirmed the ability of *Candida* to proliferate in protein hydrolysate TPN solutions, generally more rapidly than bacteria.

2.1.2.4 *Summary of* in vitro *studies*

Minor discrepancies between studies in results with similar species and similar fluids are probably related to microbial strain differences and as previously noted, variations in study design, yet the 14 published studies

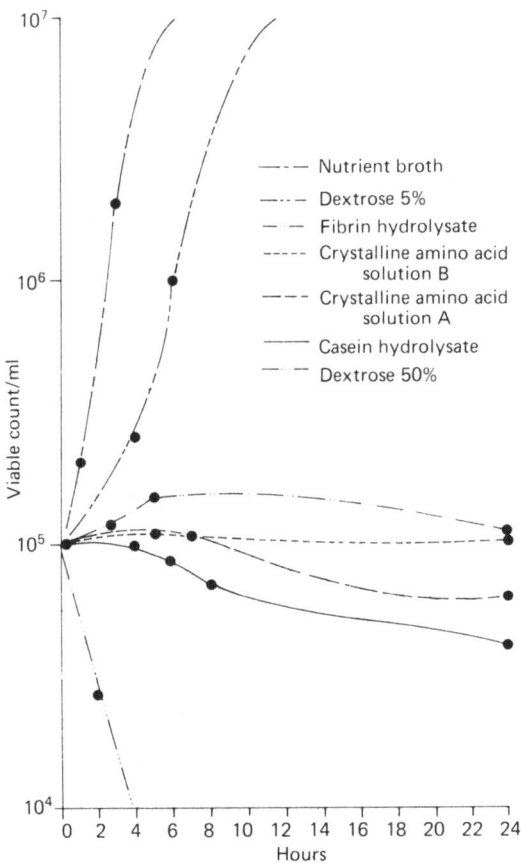

Figure 2.3 Growth of *Ps. cepacia* in various solutions for infusion at 37 °C. (From Gelbart *et al.*[18], courtesy of *Appl. Microbiol.*)

TABLE 2.5 Growth of microbial pathogens in commercial solutions for intravenous infusion*

Solution	Published study	Microorganism				
		Staph.†	Enterococcus	Esch. coli	Proteus	Ps. aeruginosa
Dextrose 5%	15, 17, 18	0	0	0	0	0
Distilled water	16, 27, 28	0				+ + + +
Dextrose 10%	16	0				0
Normal saline	5, 15–17	0		0	0	0
Dextrose 5% in saline	16, 19, 20	0	0	+ +		0
Ringer's lactate	16, 17, 19	0		+		+ +
Dextrose 5% in Ringer's	17	0		0		0
Dextrose 50%	16, 18	0		0		0
8·5–10% Amino acids in 5% dextrose	18–20	0	+ + +	0	0	0
Amino acids in 50% dextrose	25	0		0		0
10% Casein hydrolysate in 50% dextrose	22–26	+ + + +		+ + + +	+ + + +	0
10% Lipid emulsion	16	0–+ + + +	+	+ + + +	+ +	+ + + +

Table 2.5 (continued)

Solution	Published study	Ps. cepacia	Microorganism — Tribe Klebsielleae Klebsiellea	Tribe Klebsielleae Enterobacter	Tribe Klebsielleae Serratia	Acinetobacter	Candida
Dextrose 5%	15, 17, 18	++++	++++	++++	++++	0-+	+
Distilled water	16, 27, 28	++++	0		++		0
Dextrose 10%	16	+	0		+		0
Normal saline	5, 15-17	0	0-++	0-+	0-+	0-+	0
Dextrose 5% in saline	16, 19, 20	0	+	++	0-+		
Ringer's lactate	16, 17, 19		0	++	++	0	
Dextrose 5% in Ringer's	17		+	+		+	
Dextrose 50%	16, 18	0	0	0	0		0
8·5-10% Amino acids in 5% dextrose	18-20	0	0	0-++	0-+		++
Amino acids in 50% dextrose	25		0	0	0		++‡
10% Casein hydrolysate in 50% dextrose	22-26		++++	++++	++++		++‡
10% Lipid emulsion	16**	++++	++++	++++	++++	++++	++

*0 = no growth or die off at 25 °C over 24-48 hours
  + = 1 log growth at 25 °C over 24-48 hours
 ++ = 2 logs growth at 25 °C over 24-48 hours
+++ = 3 logs growth at 25 °C over 24-48 hours
++++ = 4 logs growth at 25 °C over 24-48 hours

Blank = adequate published data not available.
† Growth properties of Staph. aureus and Staph. epidermidis are very similar
‡ T. glabrata possesses similar growth properties
** Maki, D. G. and Sarafin, H. Unpublished study

are in general concurrence. Table 2.5 summarizes the results of these studies of growth of over 250 strains representing 11 genera in 12 of the most heavily utilized commercial products for infusion. Most of these studies were carried out at 25 °C. Growth in D5%/W is limited almost exclusively to members of the tribe Klebsielleae and *Ps. cepacia* (Figure 2.3); in normal saline, where growth is much poorer, to tribe Klebsielleae organisms; in distilled water to pseudomonads (Figures 2.4 and 2.5) and

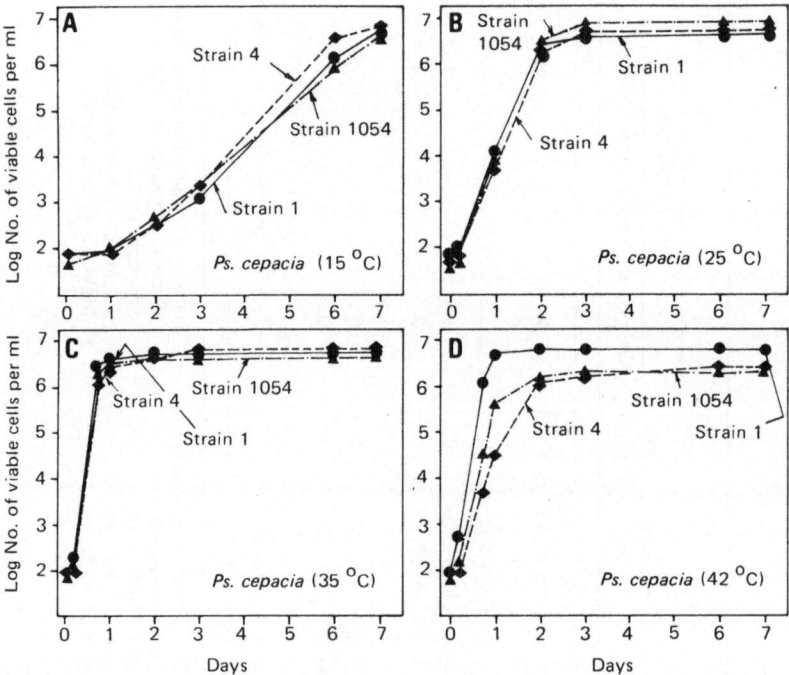

Figure 2.4 Comparative growth of three strains of *Ps. cepacia* in distilled water at 15 °C, 25 °C, 35 °C and 42 °C. (From Carson *et al.*[28], courtesy of *Appl. Microbiol.*)

Serratia; and in lactated Ringer's solution to *Ps. aeruginosa*, *Enterobacter* and *Serratia*. Much less growth (mainly of scattered Gram-negative bacilli) is supported by 5% dextrose in lactated Ringer's solution or 5% dextrose in saline. None of the tested strains grow in 50% dextrose. In contrast, virtually all except *Ps. aeruginosa* multiply rapidly in casein hydrolysate in 50% dextrose, yet growth in an amino acid solution in 50% dextrose is limited to *Candida albicans* and *Torulopsis*. Staphylococci grow in none of the 11 solutions except casein hydrolysate in 50% dextrose; *Enterococcus* multiplies only in an $8\cdot5\%$ synthetic amino acid solution in 5% dextrose. We have recently found that except for *S. epidermis* and enterococcus, all other of 13 bacterial species and *Candida* tested grew rapidly in a commercial lipid emulsion for infusion (Maki, D. G. and Sarafin, H. Unpublished study).

Growth in D5%/W or the other conventional solutions that support growth generally plateaus at approximately 10^6 organisms per ml; visible signs of microbial presence have been almost invariably absent with bacteria[2,5,15,17,27,28]. In contrast, growth of both bacteria and yeasts in casein hydrolysate-dextrose solutions produces overt turbidity within 48 hours[22,23,25,26].

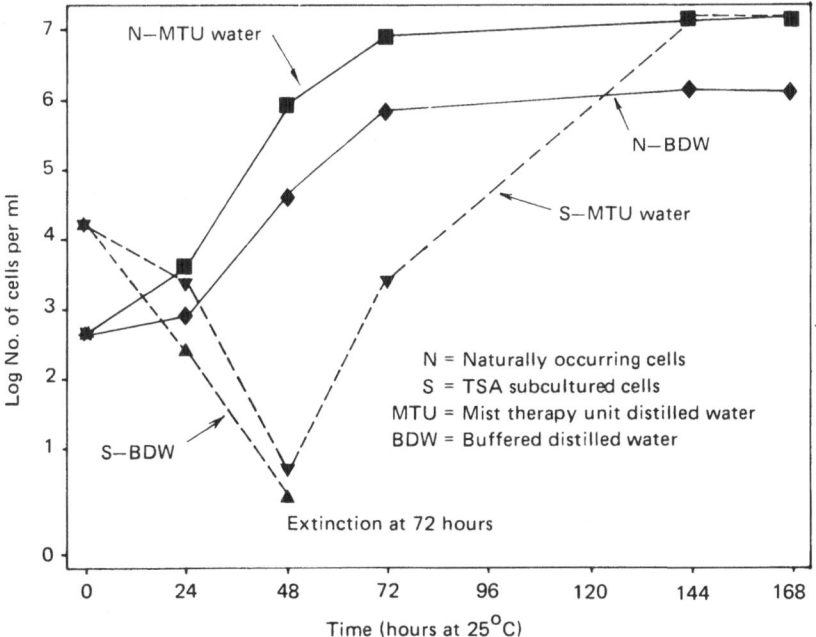

Figure 2.5 Growth of *Ps. aeruginosa* in distilled water at 25 °C; effect of subculturing naturally occurring strains is apparent. (From Favero *et al.*[27], courtesy of *Appl. Microbiol.*)

Some bacteria which grow very poorly if at all over 24–48 hours of incubation will eventually reach logarithmic growth and concentrations exceeding 10^3 per ml after many days, weeks or even months of incubation[16,17,19,25–27,30]; turbidity may then become apparent[30]. However, except for those rare instances of long standing intrinsic contamination of fluid[30,31], it is unlikely that these slow-growing organisms pose much of a hazard to the hospitalized patient receiving infusion therapy. In over 90% of reports of septicaemia traced to contaminated conventional parenteral fluids, microorganisms able to proliferate rapidly in the involved solutions have been implicated[2,4–8,11,12,29–31a].

2.1.3 Microbial physiology of growth in infusion fluid

Microbial physiologists have long been aware of the wide range in nutritional requirements and adaptability to environmental extremes among the various microbial species[32,33], reaffirmed in these studies. Commercially available D5%/W might be characterized at first glance as a relative minimal microbiological medium. It is acidic with a pH range of $3 \cdot 5$ to $5 \cdot 5$[34] and contains only dissolved atmospheric N_2 as nitrogen source; glucose and dissolved CO_2 provide the sole sources of carbon. Trace amounts of inorganic elements such as manganese, zinc and copper have been demonstrated in commercial infusion fluids[35]. *E. aerogenes* is able to utilize free nitrogen[13], and other members of tribe Klebsielleae isolated from the intestine of man, especially *E. cloacae*, have been reported by Bergerson and Hipsley to have nitrogen-fixing capabilities[36]. Mahl and his co-workers were able to demonstrate nitrogen fixation in 42% of *Kl. pneumoniae* strains among 61 tribe Klebsielleae strains tested[37]. Although some pseudomonads also can incorporate free nitrogen[38] and strains of *Ps. aeruginosa* have been shown not only to subsist but actually proliferate in tap and even distilled water[27] (Figure 2.5), some property of D5%/W or lack of one or more needed nutrients is inhibitory. In our study[15], none of the ten *Ps. aeruginosa* strains grew. Inability of *Pseudomonas*, *Proteus* and three of the four *Acinetobacter* strains to grow in D5%/W was not anticipated since these organisms are common nosocomial pathogens which are frequently encountered in a free living state in the inanimate hospital environment.

Favero, *et al.*[27] found that 'naturally occurring' strains of *Ps. aeruginosa*, obtained from water sources in the hospital, inoculated directly into distilled water without prior subculture in growth medium, multiplied rapidly whereas strains precultured in broth prior to inoculation grew poorly (Figure 2.5). It is unlikely that this phenomenon obtains in our study or those of others despite an unavoidable logistic necessity to preculture test strains; i.e. these *in vitro* studies are indeed clinically relevant:

1. During the 1970–71 US nationwide outbreak, 22 microbial species— most non-Klebsielleae—were ultimately recovered from intrinsically

contaminated Abbott cap assemblies[7, 8], yet nearly all clinical infections were caused by tribe Klebsielleae organisms[4-6, 8].

2. In surveys during this period, a wide variety of 'naturally occurring' organisms, again many non-Klebsielleae, were isolated from Abbott, Baxter and Cutter infusions sampled during clinical use, yet with rare exception only members of the tribe Klebsielleae were present in concentrations suggesting multiplication (> 10 organisms per ml)[4, 8-10].

We did not attempt to define categorically the specific biochemical factors inhibiting growth of non-Klebsielleae strains in D5%/W. Preliminary experiments suggest that the acidic pH is the primary deterrent to growth of *Pseudomonas* and *Acinetobacter* and both adverse pH and deficiencies of required nutrients or growth factors inhibit staphylococci and non-Klebsielleae Enterobactereaciae. Despite the fact that many members of the tribe Klebsielleae are facultative pychrophiles[14, 39] and grow well at 25 °C, it is unlikely that temperature significantly influenced growth of other organisms in this study, especially of *Pseudomonas*, *Acinetobacter*, *Proteus*, *Esch. coli* or *Candida*. That staphylcocci require extrinsic thiamine and uracil[32] probably explains at least in part the absolute inability of staphylcoccal strains to multiply in these fluids. Although it has been speculated that *Candida* might be capable of fixing atmospheric nitrogen, reported requirements for potassium and probably specific amino acids and vitamins[40] probably prevents growth in D5%/W or even 50% dextrose in water. *Candida* does proliferate in both solutions if amino acids or peptides are added. Environments more acidic and more minimal in terms of nutrients than needed for optimal growth have been shown to promote survival of starved microbial populations[41-43]; many of these solutions meet these conditions.

Ewing has recently proposed inclusion of the *herbicola–lathyri* group of *Erwinia* in the tribe Klebsielleae, genus *Enterobacter*, as a new species *E. agglomerans*[3]. Selective growth properties of *Erwinia* strains in D5%/W demonstrated in our study, comparable with strains of *Klebsiella*, other *Enterobacter* species and *Serratia* lends support to this taxonomic classification.

2.1.4 Clinical and epidemiological implications

As noted, despite the fact that over 22 microbial species were ultimately isolated from Abbott's elastomer-lined closures in the 1970–71 US outbreak[7, 8], nearly all clinical infections were caused by members of the tribe Klebsielleae, *E. cloacae*, *E. agglomerans*, and *Kl. pneumoniae*[4-6, 8], consistent with the selective growth properties of this tribe in glucose-containing fluids for infusion. Tribe Klebsielleae organisms might accordingly be predicted to predominate in the glucose-rich environment of the infusion product manufacturing plant. Forty-eight (50%) of ninety-six environmental cultures examined from the Rocky Mount, North Carolina, Abbott facility in March 1971, yielded Klebsielleae strains[7]. Similarly, these organisms predominated in the plant environment[44] as well as in infections[30] linked to contaminated infusion fluid in the Devonport outbreak.

Conventional infusion fluids of many types but particularly D5%/W is clearly an excellent growth medium for many ubiquitous microbial pathogens. If these *in vitro* data had been available, fluid could long ago have been predicted to be a significant potential source of nosocomial septicaemia. Since 1970, six outbreaks[11,12,29-31a] besides the US nationwide epidemic, including two in Great Britain[29,30], have been traced to contaminated crystalloids for infusion. Members of the tribe Klebsielleae were implicated in 22 of the 28 cases in 5 incidents[11,12,30-31a]. *Citrobacter freundii* caused 3 cases of septicaemia in a small outbreak traced to intrinsically contaminated 5% dextrose in lactated Ringer's solution[31]; as might be expected the epidemic strains of *Citrobacter* were found to multiply rapidly in this specific product. In the single epidemic of intravenous fluid-related sepsis in which organisms of the Klebsielleae did not predominate[29], *Ps. thomasii* infections were linked to contaminated distilled water used to cool infusion bottles after autoclaving. *Pseudomonas cepacia*, which *Ps. thomasii* resembles, multiplies rapidly in distilled water[28] and also appears to be one of the rare, non-Klebsielleae species capable of rapid growth in D5%/W[18]. Recently, outbreaks of *E. cloacae*, *Ps. cepacia*, *Ps. acidivorans*, *Flavobacter* and *E. cloacae* septicaemia have been traced to arterial pressure monitoring apparatus[45-48]. In three outbreaks extrinsic contamination of pressure transducers was presumably transmitted to the patient in the heparinized saline solutions utilized in these monitoring systems[45,47,48].

Excluding the occasional outbreaks linked to intrinsic contamination, most contamination of infusion fluid is probably extrinsic. Reported rates of in-use contamination range from 0·9 to 38% and generally average about 5%[1,9,10,12] (see Chapter 8). Organisms are introduced during manipulations of the system required to prepare it for use and during administration of fluid to the patient. Tribe Klebsielleae organisms are among the most frequently recovered Gram-negative bacilli from hands of both hospital personnel[50,51] and patients[52]. Rates of fluid contamination in use are directly proportional to the duration of uninterrupted infusion therapy[1,9,10,12]. Once introduced into a running infusion, microorganisms capable of growth in fluid can perpetuate for days in the delivery tubing despite serial replacements of the bottle[1,2].

These data indicate that parenteral infusions are at definite risk of becoming contaminated during hospital use. Contamination by micro-organisms poses an increased hazard because of their ability to rapidly proliferate in fluid, such as Klebsielleae in D5%/W. Taking into account the cumulative nature of in-use contamination of fluid and the explosive growth potential of certain microorganisms, solutions should be used immediately after compounding. Furthermore, replacing all bottles and delivery apparatus every 24–48 hours and at each change of cannula should confer protection against contamination of fluid, both of extrinsic and intrinsic origin. This preventive measure alone decreased the rate of septicaemia caused by intrinsically contaminated products during the US epidemic in 1970–71, although obviously did not totally curtail these infections[4–6,8]. Periodic set change and the use of in-line membrane microbial filters (less than 0·45 micron pore size) are the primary specific measures for reducing the hazard of contaminated fluids.

Routine buffering of inherently acidic solutions by adding sodium bicarbonate immediately before use has been advocated to diminish the incidence of infusion phlebitis[53]. We found that neutralization of D5%/W to pH 7·34 alone permits rapid growth of *Pseudomonas* and *Acinetobacter* in addition to Klebsielleae. Widening the spectrum of microorganisms capable of growth in fluid and the added risk of introducing contaminants with extra manipulations argue against routine neutralization before use.

Minute quantities of blood (1 : 500 by volume) in glucose-containing solutions also buffer fluid[54], besides providing organic nutrients for fastidious organisms otherwise incapable of growth in fluid. Moreover, blood products are a source of introduced organisms, often members of the tribe Klebsielleae[55]. Thus, following administration of blood products the entire delivery apparatus should be replaced.

Inability to detect visually microbial growth in conventional infusion fluid, even with counts exceeding 10^6 per ml in most studies, is noteworthy and may be related to the markedly reduced size of microorganisms in these fluids[28]. Inspection of the bottle and delivery apparatus when it is set up and thereafter is strongly recommended to identify mechanical abnormalities such as cracks, leaks, or particulate matter and it may occasionally reveal turbidity or other abnormalities denoting heavy bacterial contamination as occurred in the Devonport incident[30] and in the outbreak with *Cl. freundii* in the US[31]. However, in the vast majority of reports linking sepsis to contaminated fluid, including the hundreds of cases in the US outbreak in 1970–71, visible evidence of microbial presence was not noted despite often heavy contamination[2,4–6,8,11,12,29,31a, 45–49]. Hence, inspection *cannot* be relied upon to detect bacterial contamination of conventional infusion fluid. Moulds introduced through breaks in the container may produce faint turbidity or filmy precipitates[56,57].

In the past 15 years there has been a progressive and steep increase in nosocomial septicaemias caused by members of the tribe Klebsielleae, especially *Klebsiella, Enterobacter* and *Serratia*[58-62]. This has generally been attributed to ever-increasing use of antimicrobial drugs selecting for these resistant pathogens. However, the use of infusion therapy has also expanded tremendously in recent years. Accordingly, the increasing frequency of tribe Klebsielleae blood stream infections might be related in part to a rising incidence of fluid-related septicaemia, most cases unrecognized as due to contaminated fluids, or simply ascribed to the cannula.

Clinical and epidemiological translation of the *in vitro* growth abilities of *Candida* in solutions for TPN is less clear than of growth studies of bacteria in conventional infusion fluids. With the exception of one report[23], *Candida* has not commonly been recovered from culture surveys of in-use TPN fluid and septicaemia arising from such contamination has been rare[22,63]. More likely these fluids promote *Candida*'s selective multiplication in the thrombus which envelops the intravenous catheter.

2.2 METHODS FOR DETECTION OF MICROORGANISMS IN FLUIDS FOR INFUSION

2.2.1 Microbiological methods

2.2.1.1 *Bases for microbiological sampling of infusion fluid*

Microbiological sampling of fluid usually has one of two goals, in prevention as part of a programme of quality control, either in the hospital or in the manufacturing plant or in diagnosis, to identify contamination suggested by the physical appearance of an infusion system (for instance, turbidity), the clinical picture, (for instance, sepsis of indeterminate origin), or epidemiological data (for instance, a cluster of primary septicaemias). Because sampling programmes, particularly if large-scale such as those used in quality control monitoring, are technically demanding and expensive, it is important first to examine critically the indications for and appropriateness of sampling.

(a) *During manufacture.* Preventing contamination during the manufacture of infusion products remains a challenge for industry and regulatory agencies. Four outbreaks arising from intrinsically contaminated products in the US and Great Britain since 1970[4-8,29-31] attest to this fact and point to inadequacies in existent programmes of quality control. Although current USP regulations[64] now specify microbiological testing of up to

500 ml of the contents of a large volume parenteral (LVP), rather than the minute 10 ml required up until 1972, only 10–20 units from each production batch of 5–10 000 units are required to be sampled. Microbiological identification of recovered contaminants beyond Gram-stain morphology is not mandatory nor is testing of the finished products. (Abbott in 1970, along with other manufacturers, sampled bottles at an intermediate stage of production, immediately after autoclaving; contamination occurred later in production[7].) Moreover, USP does not yet require companies to use the history of prior quality control microbiological testing in judging the sterility of subsequent production; it does not even require the company to report results of sampling to a central agency.

Since 1972, officials in the US Food and Drug Administration have maintained that because contamination is such a low frequency event, product sterility testing by microbiological sampling is a statistically inadequate means of certifying product sterility[65]. Rather, 'good manufacturing practices' which, as they apply to sterility, emphasize microbiological control of presterilization manufacturing procedures, and liberal use of biological indicators and chemical–physical sterilization monitors (for instance, centrally placed thermocouples in the autoclave), are considered more important and valuable. They have exerted little, if any, effort to upgrade sampling programmes in the industry and question its necessity altogether.

This viewpoint is shortsighted, because it totally disregards the fact that three of the four outbreaks caused by intrinsically contaminated large-volume parenterals were not due to inadequacy of the sterilization process, but were due to *post*-sterilization contamination[7,29,31]. Microbiological sampling of the *finished* product is the only hope of detecting this type of contamination arising from unexpected and often unpredictable circumstances.

It is admittedly impossible to be strongly confident of the sterility of any individual batch unless a prohibitively large sample of units is examined[65]. However, sequential sampling schemes which utilize results of all prior testing in judging the sterility of a given batch can clearly identify deviation from the baseline. The level of intrinsic contamination of fluid with epidemic pathogens in the two US outbreaks was approximately 6 per 1000 bottles[7,8,31]. A sequential sampling programme which screened 1 of every 100 units produced (i.e., 100 units per 10 000 unit load) would probably have detected this level of intrinsic contamination of Abbott's products in 1970–71 within several weeks rather than the 6 months (and hundreds of cases of human illness) which were ultimately required for its discovery[7,66,66a].

Low-level contamination, even when relatively frequent, may be missed unless a significant fraction or all of the fluid in the container is cultured. The value of microbiological sampling can also be greatly enhanced by identifying contaminants at least to the genus level. Gram-negative bacilli should routinely be speciated to identify organisms with growth potential in these fluids. Such a procedure would derive meaningful information about the microbiological safety of the manufacturing processes. One isolation of an organism able to grow in the fluid tested or of a common organism from several units, even in the absence of reports of clinical infection, would prompt an intensive review of the manufacturing process. Integral features of a more optimal product sterility testing programme in industry which seem clearly warranted on the basis of past experiences are contained in Table 2.6. Obviously, microbiological sampling must not replace meticulous monitoring of the sterilization process by centrally placed and accurate recording thermocouples and biological indicators[65] but sampling should complement such monitoring.

TABLE 2.6   Features of product sterility testing during manufacturing which can greatly increase its value

1. *Sampling of finished products*, when newly-produced stock reaches the warehouse (rather than at an intermediate stage of production)

2. *Total-volume* sampling (rather than fractions)

3. *Direct addition of hyperconcentrated broth* to the container (rather than membrane filtration)

4. *More sensitive culture media* such as enriched (0·5% beef extract) brain-heart infusion broth (rather than thioglycolate media)

5. *Complete microbiological identification (to species level)* of all recovered isolates from positive quality control specimens, especially of Gram-negative bacilli

6. *Sequential sampling programmes* which utilize the results of prior testing in making judgements as to the sterility of a given batch

7. *Reporting of results* of all sterility testing in the industry to a central monitoring agency

(b) *In the hospital*. The necessity for routine quality control sampling of parenteral products within hospitals is unknown and controversial at the present time. A number of institutions in the United States have developed sophisticated sampling programmes which carry out total-volume sampling and statistically define an 'acceptable' baseline rate of contamination[67-70] (Figure 2.6). Most of these programmes sample admixtures immediately after preparation in the central pharmacy before distribution to patient care units[67,68]; solutions compounded for TPN are most frequently monitored. However, some hospitals monitor in-use contamination by sampling fluid taken directly from patients' infusions[69,70]. In both types of programmes, rates of contamination have generally been quite low, ranging from 0·9 to 5·2%.

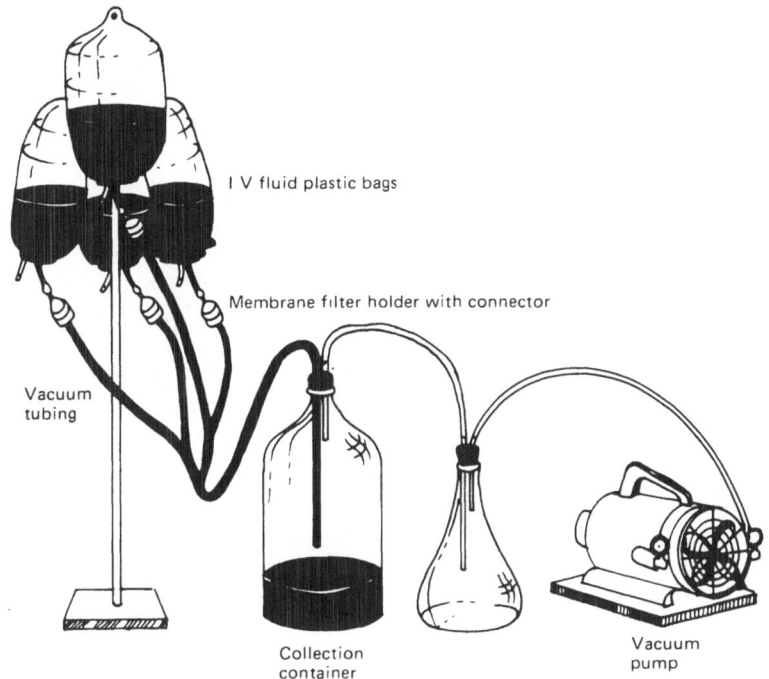

Figure 2.6 One US hospital's system for sampling infusion fluids by membrane filtration after pharmacy preparation. (From Buth *et al.*[67], courtesy of *Drug Intell. Clin. Pharm.*)

No hospital programme to date has reported identifying a problem which could pose a hazard to patients. Such sampling is probably most effective for reinforcing in personnel the need for stringent adherence to aseptic technique during preparation and administration of parenteral solutions[70]. But, considering the inadequacy of current USP recommendations for product sterility monitoring by the manufacturer, these in-hospital programmes might also be of value as a secondary screen—albeit uncomfortably close to the patient—against intrinsically contaminated products. But, viewing the low level of intrinsic contamination of fluid in the two US outbreaks (approximately 6 per 1000 units) one can question whether the relatively limited numbers of units sampled by any single intramural programme could detect a manufacturing problem of this degree. Because intrinsic contamination of closures by epidemic pathogens was far more frequent (8·1 %)[7,8], a very modest intrahospital programme of sampling of in-use fluid might well have detected the Abbott problem. A comparative study of 135 Abbott and 148 Cutter infusion systems, sampled during use in one hospital in February 1971 showed an eight-fold greater rate of contamination of Abbott systems by (epidemic) pathogens with growth potential in fluid (Table 2.7). Current intramural hospital sampling programmes might conceivably detect future problems with intrinsically contaminated infusion products.

TABLE 2.7   Comparative study of Abbott and Cutter infusions during use in one hospital during 1970–71 US outbreak traced to intrinsic contamination of Abbott infusion products*

Categories	Brand†	
	Abbott	Cutter
Number of infusion systems sampled‡	135	148
Number of contaminated systems	27	10
(%)	(20·0)	(6·8)
Number of systems contaminated with:		
E. cloacae	5	1
E. agglomerans (Erwinia)	3	0
Kl. pneumoniae	2	1
Total, tribe Klebsielleae	8	1
(%)	(5·8)	(0·7)
Number 'heavily' contaminated (>100 organisms/infusion)	7	1

* Maki, D. G., Sher, N. and Mandell, G. Unpublished data
† Patients received one or the other brand by random allocation; all systems sampled during clinical use in the hospital
‡ By membrane filtration of remaining contents of bottles and administration sets

If hospitals manufacture their own parenteral fluids, they should be required to have the same comprehensive programmes for sterility monitoring as commercial manufacturers, including microbiological sampling of the product. And lastly, infusion products found defective on physical grounds or suspected of causing clinical illness should also be sampled by the hospital. Methods for such sampling are described below.

2.2.1.2 *Environment for optimal sampling*

Except for a clever, recently reported method for product sterility testing[71], culturing of LVPs almost invariably requires manipulation of large volumes of culture media and the fluid to be tested, providing ample opportunity for entry of sampling contaminants. Because the rate of fluid contamination in manufacturers' sterility testing programmes and even in intrahospital programmes of quality control is generally quite low, ranging from much less than 1% to approximately 5%, sampling contamination can be devastating. Sampling optimally should be performed under the most stringent conditions of environmental sterility, particularly striving to control airborne and contact contamination. Within the manufacturing plant where one positive unit can force destruction of a batch of many thousand units, environmental control has taken on a space-age aura including extreme degrees of air control and total body jumpsuits, masks and sterile gloves. Within the hospital such extreme measures are not feasible nor are they probably necessary. However, sampling in the hospital should ideally be performed in a laminar flow hood which is regularly monitored. If this is not available, use of a minimally occupied laboratory is acceptable; a facemask and sterile gloves should be employed.

2.2.1.3 *Membrane filtration*

There are basically two methods for microbiological sampling, qualitative and quantitative. Except for sampling of in-use fluid suspected of harbouring large numbers of microorganisms, classic pour plate or most-probable-number methods are impractical and too insensitive to detect the low concentrations of microorganisms usually found in large volumes of contaminated fluid. Thus, membrane filtration (MF) is the most practical and well-defined technique for quantifying contamination. Since 1971 it has been the US standard for monitoring contamination of water products[72].

At the Center for Disease Control, we began sampling fluids from LVPs by MF in 1970. The volume to be sampled (usually the entire volume) is drawn under negative pressure through a membrane filter (0·22 or 0·45-micron pore size). The filter is then placed on the premoistened surface (1 drop of broth) of a sheep's blood agar plate, and incubated for 48 hours at 35–37 °C and then at room temperature for 5 days. All colonies appearing on the membrane are enumerated and microbiologically identified (Figure 2.7). Specific details of this sampling procedure have been published[7,8,10].

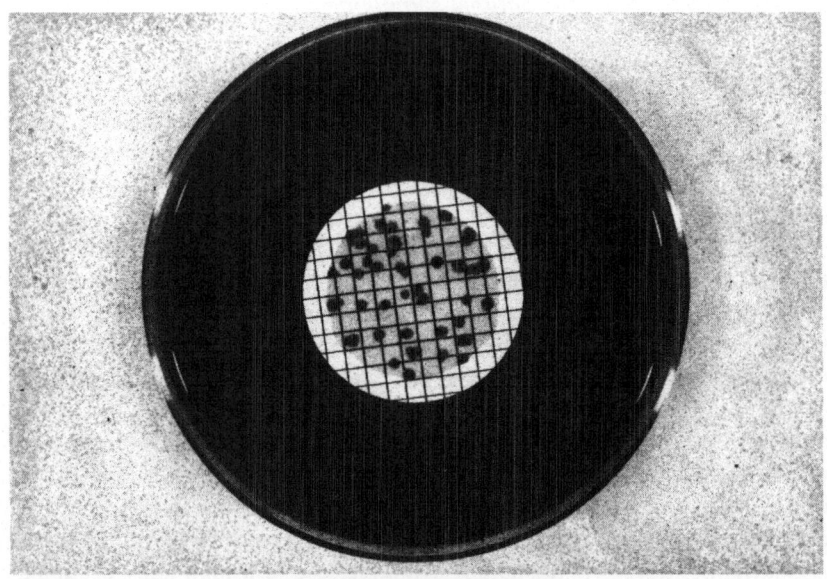

Figure 2.7 Colonies of *Ps. aeruginosa* obtained by the quantitative membrane filtration (MF) method of culturing infusion fluid.

2.2.1.4 *Qualitative methods*

(a) *Hyperconcentrated broth method.* In general, although quantitation of contamination is ideal, it is probably unnecessary. Confirming the presence of microorganisms capable of growth in fluid (such as members of the tribe Klebsielleae or pseudomonads) or identifying contamination with the same organisms simultaneously isolated from the patient's blood is clearly of greater importance. Sensitivity should supersede quantitation in choice of sampling methods.

We have found the introduction of two- to eleven-fold hyperconcentrated enriched (0·5% beef extract) brain–heart infusion broth (EBHIB) directly into the fluid container is a simple and highly sensitive method for detecting ultra-low-level contamination of fluid[7,8]. Inoculated containers are incubated at 35–37 °C for 7 days. All containers are inspected daily and any showing visible evidence of growth are subcultured to blood agar and McConkey agar plates for microbiological identification. We found this technique to be clearly superior to the MF technique described above in a comparative study of 107 one-litre bottles sampled under

TABLE 2.8 Comparative study of direct addition of hyper-concentrated broth and membrane filtration techniques for culturing infusion fluid*

| | Number of bottles positive | |
Results with method†	Any organism	Epidemic organism
Positive only by broth	17	5
Positive only by membrane filtration	0	0
Positive by both techniques	25	0
Negative by both techniques	65	102

* Mackel et al.[7]
† One litre bottles samples; one-half of contents sampled by membrane filtration and remaining 500 ml by adding double-strength enriched (0.5% beef extract) brain–heart infusion broth (EBHIB)

strict conditions of asepsis in a laminar flow hood at the Center for Disease Control during the 1970–71 outbreak (Table 2.8)[7].

Rycroft and Moon[71] recently described a clever related method for sterility monitoring of LVPs by total volume culture. Dehydrated broth powder is added directly, before autoclaving, to a random sample of bottles from each batch. The test bottles are then incubated after sterilization. Although possessing advantages of simplicity and total volume sampling, intrinsic contamination of the closure is not detected. Nonetheless, a modification of the method might prove very effective and economically advantageous for industry.

(b) *USP method.* The USP currently specifies a qualitative MF method for LVPs[64], but directs aseptically cutting the membrane in two and immersing one-half in 100 ml of thioglycolate medium for incubation at 30–35 °C and the other half into 100 ml of soya-bean–casein digest medium (trypticase soy broth) for incubation at 20–25 °C. Both media are incubated for at least 7 days. Whether this technique is more sensitive than the quantitative MF method or more important, is as sensitive as addition of hyperconcentrated broth to the container is unknown. The USP method clearly requires more manipulations and is technically more demanding than use of hyperconcentrated broth.

2.2.1.5 *Method for culturing suspect in-use fluid in the hospital‡*

When it is necessary to sample in-use fluid suspected of harbouring contaminants, the specific type of fluid and its exact lot number should be

‡ For recommendations from the DHSS in the UK see HSC(IS) 118 and 119, March 1975

TABLE 2.9   Method for culturing suspect in-use fluid in the hospital*

1. Record the nature of the fluid and all lot numbers

2. Cap the administration set with a sterile enclosed needle and transport promptly to the laboratory in a clean plastic bag. Sampling should be done in a clean, minimally occupied laboratory, in a laminar flow hood if possible

3. Withdraw 10–20 ml of fluid from the administration (drip) set:
   (a) Culture $0 \cdot 1$ (surface) or $1 \cdot 0$ ml (pour plate) quantitatively in solid medium
   (b) Inject remaining fluid into a blood culture bottle

4. Add an equal volume of double concentrated EBHIB† to remaining fluid in the container—or if the container is empty add 50 ml and swirl —and incubate the container
   (Fluid from the container may also be first cultured quantitatively as in 3(a))

5. Attempt to obtain and culture remaining samples of any other fluids the patient may have received in the preceding 24–48 hours

6. Incubate all containers at 35–37 °C for at least 7 days before discarding‡

7. All isolates should be fully speciated

8. If the clinical and epidemiological data suggest contamination during manufacture (intrinsic), the public health authorities should immediately be informed. Remaining unused suspect products should not be sampled by the hospital but retained for evaluation by these agencies

---

* Modified from: Septicemias associated with contaminated intravenous fluid. In *National Nosocomial Infections Study.* Quarterly Report, Second Quarter of 1972, (Atlanta, Georgia: US Public Health Service)
† Enriched (0·5% beef extract) brain–heart infusion broth (EBHIB)
‡ If contaminated blood products are suspected, specimens should also be incubated at 27 °C

carefully recorded (Table 2.9). In addition, an attempt should be made to determine the nature and lot numbers of all other fluids and intravenous medications the patient has received in the preceding 24–48 hours.

A sterile closure (a sterile ensheathed needle works very well) should be placed on the end of the administration tubing and the entire system transported to the laboratory in a plastic bag for immediate culture. Ten to 20 ml of fluid can be withdrawn from the line with a syringe: and $0 \cdot 1$ ml spread on the surface of a blood agar plate or 1 ml incorporated into a conventional trypticase soy agar pour plate. The remaining fluid is inoculated directly into a blood culture bottle. If only qualitative screening is desired initially, 5–10 ml can be refrigerated for future quantitation.

Fluid from the container can also be cultured first quantitatively as described above. Then if the fluid container is more than half full, drain to half full aseptically and add to the container an equal volume of double-strength EBHIB. Smaller quantities of fluid may be cultured by adding 50 ml of broth and swirling the container. Cultures should be incubated for at least 7 days before being discarded as negative. All isolates, which should be speciated and tested for antimicrobial susceptibility, should be saved until the scope of the problem has been elucidated.

Alternate but less sensitive techniques for culturing remaining fluid in the container are the substitution of trypticase soy broth for EBHIB or the passage of the remaining contents of the container through a 0·22-micron filter and culture of one-half of the filter on blood agar and one-half in broth (similar to the USP method).

If intrinsic contamination is suspected, all unused fluids of the implicated lot number should be retained for testing by public health laboratories. The local or state and national health authorities (in the US the Food and Drug Administration and the Center for Disease Control) should be informed immediately. It is questionable whether hospitals should attempt to culture unopened LVPs. As previously noted, the incidence of contamination, even in reported cases has often been very low and final resolution may require sampling of large volumes of unopened products. An individual hospital laboratory culturing a few samples would be unlikely to obtain meaningful results. Moreover, the implications of intrinsic contamination require unimpeachable sampling methods. Cultures are probably better performed by state or federal agencies equipped to examine a large number of samples with the most sensitive techniques and in laminar flow facilities.

2.2.1.6 Endotoxin assays

Recently two cases of contaminated infusion fluid provided an opportunity for testing the efficacy of the limulus assay for endotoxin in detecting contamination of infusate[49]. Direct assay of in-use fluid was strongly positive (testing of dilutions was not reported); however, the level of contamination was massive, exceeding 100 000 viable *Ps. aeruginosa* per ml. Although the limulus assay is a promising technique and is quite sensitive for detection of endotoxin[73], it is probably too insensitive to be of value in commercial quality control programmes; because at least 100–1000 organisms per ml must be present to give a positive assay[74]. The assay may be of adjunctive value in rapid detection of in-use contamination by very large numbers of Gram-negative bacilli, as occasionally occurs[30,31,49] or detecting non-viable pyrogens[49]. However, it should be pointed out that the test is technically demanding, is not well standardized, and is subject to considerable false-positivity[75]. Conventional methods of bacteriological culture at the present time are the most important means of identifying contamination of infusion products. Hopefully, refinements of the limulus assay, or application of other technology for detecting microbial presence such as gas chromatography or bioluminescence will eventually provide a reliable rapid non-cultural technique for the detection of this type of contamination.

2.2.2 Detection of contamination by clinical surveillance

2.2.2.1 *Rationale*

As noted above, in reference to infusion products (or any other medications), the major effort to detect intrinsic contamination should be made in the manufacturing plant, before distribution for clinical use. But surveillance of clinical infections is a proven secondary means of detecting intrinsically contaminated infusion products and is probably the most reliable means for detecting extrinsic contamination which causes disease.

2.2.2.2 *In the hospital*

(a) *Clinical.* The potential of in-use infusion fluid to harbour contamination of either extrinsic or intrinsic origin and in particular to support rapid microbial proliferation leading to catastrophic illness has been abundantly confirmed. Containers should be inspected routinely before use; though as previously noted, the absence of macroscopic abnormality does not exclude microbial contamination. More important, contaminated infusate must be suspected and excluded microbiologically in patients with un-explained sepsis, particularly when associated with shock or which is refractory to antimicrobial therapy[1,8] (and see Chapter 10). Furthermore, the identity of the blood pathogen can strongly suggest contaminated fluid as a cause of sepsis.

(b) *Microbiological.* Laboratory surveillance for illness resulting from contaminated fluid is very simple, requiring *routine* speciation of all blood isolates and collation and continuous review of the institution's experience with bacteraemia. Ideally laboratory surveillance should go hand-in-hand with clinical surveillance. In view of the rarity of blood stream infections with *E. agglomerans* or *Ps. cepacia*, one case, occurring in a patient receiving infusion therapy should prompt an immediate search for con-taminated medications or infusion products. A cluster, even as few as two cases, should prompt a full-scale investigation including culturing of in-use fluids and informing the public health authorities. A significant increase in septicaemias caused by *E. cloacae*, *Citrobacter*, other organisms of the tribe Klebsielleae, or any other microorganisms with known growth potential in infusion products should prompt search for an infusion-related aetiology. Such actions in 1973 averted a second US nationwide epidemic when intrinsic contamination of Cutter products was rapidly identified and a recall put into effect so rapidly that the outbreak was limited to five recognized cases[31]. The same perceptiveness rapidly curtailed the Devonport outbreak[30]. Laboratory surveillance alone—leading to an awareness of an increase in blood isolates of unusual organisms alerted a number of hospitals to the 1970–71 US epidemic[8].

The US National Coordinating Committee on Large Volume Parenterals has recently provided guidelines for the detection, confirmation, and particularly the reporting of problems associated with commercial products for infusion[76].

2.2.2.3 *Nationwide*

We live in an age of unprecedented communication. Products manufactured on one side of a country can be in thousands of homes or hospitals within days or even hours. This has created a potential for dissemination of poisoned or contaminated products on a scale that is sobering and which found culmination in the US in 1970–71. The fact that such an outbreak could occur is not surprising, and *the likelihood that an epidemic of similar magnitude and geographical extent could occur in the future is very real and should continuously be anticipated.*

On a national scale, outbreaks of septicaemia arising from intrinsic contamination of nationally distributed products can be exceedingly difficult to recognize if the infections are of low frequency and occur in scattered hospitals. National surveillance networks such as the CDC National Nosocomial Infections Study which carries out surveillance of nosocomial infections in a large cross section of American hospitals[77] can serve as a sentinel system for early detection of common-source epidemics. Retrospective review of the data submitted to this fledgling programme from January 1970 to July 1971 showed conclusively that hospitals using Abbott infusion products experienced a highly significant increase in incidence of enterobacter bacteraemia beginning in July 1970, (Figure 2.8) even though none of these hospitals individually identified the aetiology or was fully aware of the scope of the problem until March 1971[78]. No increase in enterobacter bacteraemia occurred in hospitals

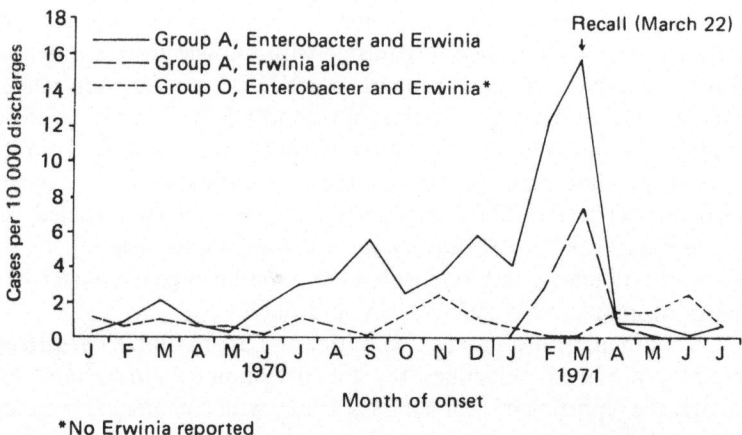

*No Erwinia reported

Figure 2.8 Primary bacteraemias caused by Erwinia and Enterobacter reported to National Nosocomial Infections Surveillance Study, US Center for Disease Control, from 37 US Hospitals between January 1970 and June 1971. A = hospitals using Abbott infusion products; O = infusion products other than Abbott's. (Nationwide Epidemic of Septicemia Associated with Intravenous Fluid Therapy: An Analysis Based on the CDC National Nosocomial Infections Study. In *National Nosocomial Infections Study*. Quarterly Report, Fourth Quarter of 1971, p. 14 (Atlanta, Georgia: US Public Health Service)

using the infusion products of other manufacturers ($p < 0.001$). Although this US surveillance programme which had its inception only in January 1970 did not detect the outbreak at its outset, the current rapidity and sophistication with which data submitted by participating hospitals is now processed would almost certainly detect a similar problem in the future.

Acknowledgements

I acknowledge and deeply appreciate the influence of a long association with Donald C. Mackel, MS and John V. Bennett, MD, friends and former colleagues at the United States Center for Disease Control, in the formulation of many of the concepts and philosophies embodied in this chapter.

References

1. Maki, D. G., Goldmann, D. A. and Rhame, F. S. (1973). Infection control in intravenous therapy. *Ann. Intern. Med.*, **79**, 867

2. Michaels, L. and Ruebner, B. (1953). Growth of bacteria in intravenous infusion fluids. *Lancet*, **i**, 772
3. Ewing, W. S. and Fife, M. A. (1971). *Enterobacter agglomerans*. The *herbicola-lathyri* bacteria. (Atlanta, Georgia: Center for Disease Control)
4. Center for Disease Control. (1971). Nosocomial bacteremias associated with intravenous fluid therapy–U.S.A. *Morbidity and Mortality Weekly Rep.*, **20** (Suppl.)
5. Felts, S. K., Shaffner, W., Melly, M. A. and Koenig, M. G. (1972). Sepsis caused by contaminated intravenous fluids: epidemiologic, clinical and laboratory investigations of an outbreak in one hospital. *Ann. Intern. Med.*, **77**, 881
6. Fisher, E. J., Maki, D. G., Eisses, J. and Quinn, E. (1971). Epidemic septicemias due to intrinsically contaminated infusion products. Abstracts of papers presented at the *Eleventh Interscience Conference for Antimicrobial Agents and Chemotherapy*, October 20, Atlantic City
7. Mackel, D. C., Maki, D. G., Anderson, R. L., Rhame, F. S. and Bennett, J. V. (1975). Nationwide epidemic of septicemia caused by contaminated intravenous products: mechanisms of intrinsic contamination. *J. Clin. Microbiol.*, **2**, 486
8. Maki, D. G., Rhame, F. S., Mackel, D. C. and Bennett, J. V. (1976). Nationwide epidemic of septicemia caused by contaminated intravenous products: epidemiologic and clinical features. *Am. J. Med.*, **60**, 471
9. Maki D. G., Rhame, F. S., Goldmann, D. A. and Mandell, G. L. (1973). The infection hazard posed by contaminated intravenous infusion fluid. *Bacteremia-Laboratory and Clinical Aspects* (Springfield, Illinois: Charles C. Thomas)
10. Maki, D. G., Anderson, R. L. and Shulman, J. A. (1974). In-use contamination of intravenous infusion fluid. *Appl. Microbiol.*, **28**, 778
11. Sack, R. A. (1970). Epidemic of Gram-negative organism septicemia subsequent to elective operation. *Am. J. Obstet. Gynecol.*, **107**, 394
12. Duma, R. J., Warner, J. F. and Dalton, H. P. (1971). Septicemia from intravenous infusions. *N. Engl. J. Med.*, **284**, 257
13. Mortenson, L. E. (1962). Inorganic nitrogen assimilation and ammonia incorporation. *The Bacteria. Vol. III. Biosynthesis.* (London and New York: Academic Press)
14. Ingraham, J. L. (1962). Temperature relationships. *The Bacteria. Vol. IV. The Physiology of Growth.* (London and New York: Academic Press)
15. Maki, D. G. and Martin, W. T. (1975). Nationwide epidemic of septicemia caused by contaminated infusion products. IV. Growth of microbial pathogens in fluids for intravenous infusion. *J. Infect. Dis.*, **131**, 267
16. Crichton, E. P. (1973). Infusion fluids as culture media. *Am. J. Clin. Pathol.*, **59**, 199
17. Guynn, J. B. Jr., Poretz, D. M. and Duma, R. J. (1973). Growth of various bacteria in a variety of intravenous fluids. *Am. J. Hosp. Pharm.*, **30**, 321
18. Gelbart, S. M., Reinhardt, G. F. and Greenlee, H. B. (1973). Multiplication of nosocomial pathogens in intravenous feeding solutions. *Appl. Microbiol.*, **26**, 874
19. Pierpaoli, P. G., Palmer, H. A. and Codino, R. J. (1973). *Drug Intell. Clin. Pharm.*, **7**, 515

20. Steckel, S. D., Gonik, M., Martens, P. J., Patel, J. A., Curtis, E. G. and Ho, N. F. (1973). *Drug. Intell. Clin. Pharm.*, **7**, 177

21. Goldmann, D. A. and Maki, D. G. (1973). Infection control in total parenteral nutrition. *J. Am. Med. Ass.*, **223**, 1360

22. Boeckman, C. R. and Krill, C. E. Jr. (1970). Bacterial and fungal infections complicating parenteral alimentation in infants and children. *J. Pediatr. Surg.*, **5**, 117

23. Deeb, E. N. and Natsios, G. A. (1971). Contamination of intravenous fluids by bacteria and fungi during preparation and administration. *Am. J. Hosp. Pharm.*, **28**, 764

24. Brennan, M. F., O'Connell, R. C., Rosol, J. A. and Kundsin, R. (1971). The growth of *Candida albicans* in nutritive solutions given parenterally. *Arch. Surg.*, **103**, 705

25. Goldmann, D. A., Martin, W. T. and Worthington, J. W. (1973). Growth of bacteria and fungi in total parenteral nutrition solutions. *Am. J. Surg.*, **126**, 314

26. Sanderson, I. and Deitel, M. (1973). Intravenous hyperalimentation without sepsis. *Surg. Gynecol. Obstet*, **136**, 577

27. Favero, M. S., Carson, L. A., Bond, W. W. and Petersen, N. J. (1971). *Pseudomonas aeruginosa*: growth in distilled water for hospitals. *Science*, **173**, 836

28. Carson, L. A., Favero, M. S., Bond, W. W. and Petersen, N. J. (1973). Morphological, biochemical, and growth characteristics of *Pseudomonas cepacia* from distilled water. *Appl. Microbiol.*, **25**, 476

29. Phillips, I., Eykyn, S. and Laker, M. (1972). Outbreak of hospital infection caused by contaminated autoclaved fluids. *Lancet*, **i**, 1258

30. Meers, P. D., Calder, M. W., Mazhar, M. M. and Lawrie, G. M. (1973). Intravenous infusion of contaminated dextrose solution. *Lancet*, **ii**, 1189

31. Center for Disease Control. (1973). Septicemias associated with contaminated intravenous fluids. *Morbidity and Mortality Weekly Report*, **22**, 99

31a. Center for Disease Control (1976). Primary Bacteremia—Illinois. *Morbidity and Mortality Weekly Report*, **25**, 110

32. Guirard, B. M. and Snell, E. E. (1962). Nutritional requirements of microorganisms. *The Bacteria. Vol. IV. The Physiology of Growth*. (London and New York: Academic Press)

33. Stokstad, E. L. R., Broquist, H. P. and Sloan, N. H. (1955). Nutrition of microorganisms. *Ann. Rev. Microbiol.*, **9**, 111

34. Lebowitz, M. H., Masuda, J. Y. and Beckerman, J. H. (1971). The pH and acidity of intravenous solutions. *J. Am. Med. Ass.*, **215**, 1937

35. James, B. E. and MacMahon, R. A. (1970). Trace elements in intravenous fluids. *Med. J. Austral.*, **2**, 1161

36. Bergersen, F. J. and Hipsley, E. H. (1970). The presence of N_2-fixing bacteria in the intestines of man and animals. *J. Gen. Microbiol.*, **60**, 61

37. Mahl, M. C., Wilson, P. W., Fife, M. A. and Ewing, W. H. (1965). Nitrogen fixation by members of the tribe Klebsielleae. *J. Bacteriol.*, **89**, 1482

38. Thimann, K. V. (1963). The life of bacteria: their growth, metabolism and relationships. (London and New York: Macmillan)

39. Wetterlow, C. H., Kay, F. H. and Edsall, G. (1954). Missed contaminations in biologic products: The role of psychrophilic bacteria. *J. Lab. Clin. Med.*, **43**, 411

40. Silardi, G. L. (1965). Nutrition of systemic and subcutaneous pathogenic fungi. *Bact. Rev.*, **29**, 406

41. Postgate, J. R. and Hunter, J. R. (1962). The survival of starved bacteria. *J. Gen. Microbiol.*, **29**, 233

42. Rose, A. H. (1965). *Chemical Microbiology*. (London: Butterworths)

43. Postgate, J. R. (1967). Viability measurements and survival of microbes under minimum stress. *Advances in Microbiologic Physiology*, Vol. 1. (London and New York: Academic Press)

44. Lapage, S. P., Johnson, R. and Holmes, B. (1973). Bacteria from intravenous fluids. *Lancet*, **ii**, 284

45. Phillips, I., Eykyn, S., Curtis, M. A. and Snell, J. J. S. (1971). *Pseudomonas cepacia* (multivorans) septicaemia in an intensive care unit. *Lancet*, **i**, 375

46. Stamm, W. E., Colella, J. J., Anderson, R. L. and Dixon, R. E. (1975). Indwelling arterial catheters as a source of nosocomial bacteremia. *N. Engl. J. Med.*, **292**, 1099

47. Center for Disease Control. (1974). Nosocomial *Pseudomonas cepacia* bacteremia caused by contaminated pressure transducers. *Morbidity and Mortality Weekly Rep.*, **23**, 423

48. Center for Disease Control. (1975). Transducer-associated bacteremia. *Morbidity and Mortality Weekly Rep.*, **24**, 295

49. Jorgensen, J. H. and Smith, R. F. (1973). Rapid detection of contaminated intravenous fluids using the *Limulus in vitro* endotoxin assay. *Appl. Microbiol.*, **26**, 521

50. Salzman, T. C., Clark, J. J. and Klemm, L. (1968). Hand contamination of personnel as a mechanism of cross-infection in nosocomial infections with antibiotic-resistant *Escherichia coli* and *Klebsiella-Aerobacter*. *Antimicrob. Agents Chemother.*, **1967**, 97

51. Knittle, M. A., Eitzman, D. V. and Baer, J. (1975). Role of hand contamination of personnel in epidemiology of Gram-negative nosocomial infections. *J. Pediatr.*, **86**, 433

52. Pollack, M., Charache, P., Nieman, R. E., Jett, M. P., Reinhardt, J. A., and Hardy, P. H. Jr. (1972). Factors influencing colonization and antibiotic-resistant patterns of Gram-negative bacteria in hospital patients. *Lancet*, **ii**, 668

53. Fonkalsrud, E. W., Pederson, B. M., Murphy, J. and Beckerman, J. H. (1968). Reduction of infusion thrombophlebitis with buffered glucose solutions. *Surgery*, **63**, 280

54. Ansel, H. C. and Gigandet, M. P. (1971). Change in pH of infusion solutions upon mixing with blood. *J. Am. Med. Ass.*, **218**, 1052

55. Braude, A. I. (1958). Transfusion reactions from contaminated blood. Their recognition and treatment. *N. Engl. J. Med.*, **258**, 1289

56. Robertson, M. H. (1970). Fungi in fluids—a hazard of intravenous therapy. *J. Med. Microbiol.*, **3**, 99

57. Maddocks, A. C. and Raine, G. (1972). Contaminated drip fluids. *Br. Med. J.*, **ii**, 231

58. Dans, P. E., Barrett, F. F., Casey, J. I. and Finland, M. (1970). *Klebsiella–Enterobacter* at Boston City Hospital. *Arch. Intern. Med.*, **125**, 94

59. Pruitt, B. A., Stein, J. M., Foley, F. D., Moncrief, J. A. and O'Neill, J. A. (1970). Intravenous therapy in burn patients-suppurative thrombophlebitis and other life-threatening complications. *Arch. Surg.*, **100**, 399

60. Finland, M. (1970). Changing ecology of bacterial infections as related to anti-bacterial therapy. *J. Infect. Dis.*, **122**, 419

61. Altemeier, W. A., McDonough, J. J. and Fullen, W. D. (1971). Third day surgical fever. *Arch. Surg.*, **103**, 158

62. Myerowitz, R. L., Medeiros, A. A. and O'Brien, T. F. (1971). Recent experience with bacillemia due to Gram-negative organisms. *J. Infect. Dis.*, **124**, 239

63. Freeman, J. B., Lemire, A. and MacLean, L. D. (1972). Intravenous alimentation and septicemia. *Surg. Gynecol. Obstet.*, **135**, 708

64. *The United States Pharmacopia.* (1975). (Easton, Pennsylvania: Mack Publishing Company)

65. Burch, C. W. (1974). Levels of sterility: probabilities of survivors vs. biological indicators. *Bull. Parenteral Drug Assoc.*, **28**, 105

66. Tenney, J., Maki, D., Rhame, F., Goldmann, D., Dixon, R. and Bennett, J. V. (1973). Intrinsic contamination of intravenous fluid products. Presented to *The* 101*st Annual Meeting of the American Public Health Association*, November, San Francisco

66a. Bennett, J. V. (1976). Minutes of the expert advisory panel on sterility control in manufacturing. National Coordinating Committee on Large Volume Parenterals, November 25, 1975

67. Buth, J. A., Coverly, R. A. and Eckel, F. M. (1973). A practical method of sterility monitoring of IV admixtures and a method of implementing a routine sterility monitoring program. *Drug Intell. Clin. Pharm.*, **7**, 276

68. Kundsin, R. B., Walter, C. W. and Scott, J. A. (1973). In-use testing of sterility of intravenous solutions in plastic containers. *Surgery*, **73**, 778

69. Hanson, A. L. and Shelley, R. M. (1974). Monitoring contamination levels of intravenous solutions using "total-sample" techniques. *Am. J. Hosp. Pharm.*, **31**, 733

70. Ravin, R., Bahr, J. *et al.* (1974). Program for bacterial surveillance of intravenous admixtures. *Am. J. Hosp. Pharm.*, **31**, 340

71. Rycroft, J. A. and Moon, D. (1975). An "in-production" method for testing the sterility of infusion fluids. *J. Hyg., Camb.*, **74**, 17

72. American Public Health Association. (1971). Standard methods for the examination of water and waste water. 13th Ed. (New York: American Public Health Association, Inc.)

73. Rojas-Corona, R. B., Skarner, R., Tamakuma, S. and Fine, J. (1969). The *Limulus* coagulation assay for endotoxin: a comparison with other assay methods. *Proc. Soc. Exp. Biol. Med.*, **132**, 599

74. Jorgensen, J. H., Carvajul, B. E., Chipps, B. E. and Smith, R. F. (1973). Rapid detection of Gram-negative bacteriuria by use of the *Limulus* endotoxin assay. *Appl. Microbiol.*, **26**, 38

75. Elin, R. J. and Wolff, S. M. (1973). Nonspecificity of the *Limulus* amebocyte lysate test: positive reactions with polynucleotides and proteins. *J. Infect. Dis.*, **128**, 349

76. US National Coordinating Committee on Large Volume Parenterals. (1975). Recommended system for surveillance and reporting of problems with large-volume parenterals in hospitals. *Am. J. Hosp. Pharm.*, **32**, 1251
77. Bennett, J. V., Scheckler, W. E., Maki, D. G. *et al.* (1971). Current national patterns, United States, *Proceedings of the International Conference on Nosocomial Infections.* (Chicago: American Hospital Association)
78. Goldmann, D. A., Fulkerson, C. C., Dixon, R. E., Maki, D. G. and Bennett, J. V. (1976). Nationwide epidemic of septicemias caused by contaminated intravenous products. II. Assessment of the problem by a National Nosocomial Infections Surveillance System. (Submitted for publication)

3

Additives—
an additional hazard?
P. F. D'Arcy

3.1 BACKGROUND INFORMATION

3.1.1 Use of intravenous infusion fluids

Intravenous infusion fluids have been in clinical use for nearly a century and a half. The first recorded intravenous infusion was given by Dr Thomas

Latta of Edinburgh during the cholera epidemic of 1832. In an attempt to save the life of an old woman patient, he injected into a vein 6 pints of water containing sodium chloride and carbonate. This infusion was administered over a period of 30 minutes. The patient died, but with constant nursing attention and frequent saline infusions, Dr Latta managed to save the lives of five out of 15 cholera victims.

Today over 10 million intravenous infusion fluids are administered each year in the United Kingdom[1], whilst the total in the United States probably exceeds 75 million[2]. Indeed the fact that so many infusions are used tends to induce a false sense of security, then tragedies are the unpleasant reminders that the hazards of intravenous infusions have not all been eliminated. For example, in the United Kingdom, some four years ago, wide publicity was given to three instances of contaminated infusion fluids, all occurring within the space of a few months.

3.1.2 Bacterial contamination

In December 1971, bacterial contamination was detected in allegedly sterile products in St Thomas's Hospital, London[3,4]. Several patients were infected, one of whom died. In March 1972, use of a batch of contaminated fluid was implicated in the deaths of six patients at Plymouth General Hospital[5,6]. The following month, a contaminated solution was detected at Kettering General Hospital when a patient suffered a non-fatal reaction[7].

It is fair to comment therefore that the present upsurge of interest and attention into all aspects of intravenous fluid manufacture and usage is a direct result of the sudden, albeit dramatic, disruption of this sense of complacency. Unfortunately sudden and dramatic accidents tend to promote 'headline-thinking' and with intravenous fluids it is vital to keep hazards or potential hazards within their correct perspective. It is salutary occasionally to recall that, although intravenous fluid therapy can be hazardous, the non-administration of such fluids to a seriously ill patient is most certainly even more hazardous.

Much useful advice has been given in the literature to encourage all associated with intravenous therapy to realize and understand their role, and the roles of others, in all stages from manufacture to use of the fluids. If any one such statement was to be selected as a general guide to good intravenous fluid practice, then most certainly it would be that given within the text of the 1973 Rosenheim Report[8], *'The safety of the patient is directly related to the understanding of essential procedures by all those involved in the handling of medicinal products . . .'*; that this statement refers to all medicinal products and not just to intravenous fluids is an additional bonus.

3.1.3 Addition of drugs to intravenous infusions

In relatively recent years, the practice of often adding multiple drugs at patient level in the ward to commercially prepared standard intravenous infusions has dramatically increased. This has raised a number of problems since there is good reason to believe that many drugs are given via the container of an intravenous infusion fluid without due regard to the stability or therapeutic integrity of such combinations[9-11]. In addition, there is a further problem associated with the addition of drugs to infusion fluids; the preservation and maintenance of the sterility of the original fluid[12].

Within the context of this Symposium it is therefore significant to note that in recent years microbial contamination has caused concern as has also drug addition to intravenous fluids. It is pertinent to ask whether circumstances exist in intravenous fluid practice where these two factors are inter-related and whether such inter-relationship (if it exists) is capable of producing a clinical hazard. It is the purpose of this paper to examine, step by step, the main facets of available evidence to determine whether or not drug additives are an additional microbiological hazard of infusion therapy.

3.2 THE EVIDENCE

3.2.1 The extent to which drug additions are made to intravenous fluids

In a survey of 10 hospitals in Ulster, carried out during a one month period in January 1972 or January 1973, D'Arcy and Thompson[10] found that of a total of 7900 separate intravenous infusions documented, 3096 (39·2%) had drugs injected into the infusion container and in a considerable proportion of these the additives were multiple. This survey also showed that ten drugs accounted for 95·8% of all the additives (Table 3.1). Other workers have since carried out similar surveys in other regions of the British Isles and it is now possible to compare these individual findings (Table 3.2). It is apparent that there is a good degree of uniformity in intravenous infusion practice throughout the British Isles. The percentage of drug additions made to intravenous fluid containers ranged from 14·3 to 44%; the common drug additives were similar in each region and most

TABLE 3.1   Percentage of drug additives to intravenous fluid containers (data from Ulster survey of
D'Arcy and Thompson[10])

Drug additive	Percentage of total
Potassium chloride	26·2
Heparin	16·7
Oxytocin and 'Syntocinon'	15·9
Lignocaine	11·0
Ampicillin	7·8
'Parentrovite'	7·6
'Imferon'	·3·3
Tetracyclines	2·8
Benzylpenicillin	2·8
'Apresoline'	1·7
Others	4·2

occurred in the 'top-ten' of the Ulster survey. Four drugs were the maximum
when multiple drug additions were made, although the number of occasions
on which these multiple additions were made showed a wide variation
between some of the regions (1·6–24%). Interestingly, Brodlie et al.[14]
working in Dundee, found that single drugs were added to fluids for
medical patients, whereas for surgical patients 15% of the additives contained two or more drugs.

The main evidence to be drawn from these surveys in the context of the
present discussion, is that the addition of drugs to the containers of
intravenous infusion fluids is a common practice throughout the hospitals
in the British Isles. A simple average calculated from the data given in
these surveys, shows that this common practice occurs overall with almost
30% of intravenous infusion fluids.

3.2.2   Theoretical calculation of potential unwanted sequelae due to drug addition to intravenous infusions

The number of infusion fluids used annually in the United Kingdom is
known (approximately 10 million), and the extent to which drug additions
are made to the fluids is established (approximately 30%). Therefore it
becomes a relatively simple exercise to project the available data, on a
purely theoretical basis, to obtain a figure for the total potential risk of
unwanted sequelae due to drug addition. These calculations are as
follows:

TABLE 3.2 Comparison of data from recent drug additive surveys

Authors	Number of infusions with additives (%)	Common drug additives	Multiple drug additives. (%)	Maximum number
D'Arcy and Thompson[10] Ulster	39·2	KCl Heparin Oxytocin Lignocaine Ampicillin	1·6	4
Hughes[13] Kent	14·3	—	3·4	3
Brodlie, Henney and Wood[14] Dundee	*	KCl Ampicillin Cephaloridine Tetracycline	Medical 0 Surgical 15	4
Harrison and Lowe[15] London	44·0†	KCl Heparin Comp. Vitamins Ampicillin	17–24	4
Timoney and Harte[16] Eire	21·2	KCl Ampicillin Hydrocortisone Heparin	—	—

* 15% incompatibilities recorded overall
† Three cases of incompatibility recorded

(i) Ten million intravenous infusion fluids are administered each year in the United Kingdom.

(ii) On average 30% of these fluids contain at least one drug additive.

(iii) Potassium chloride is the most common drug additive; (up to 50% of the total additives); however, some commercially prepared infusion fluids have now been formulated to contain potassium chloride as an intrinsic ingredient. Therefore excluding the maximum use of potassium chloride, approximately 1·5 million fluids are administered in combination with at least one other drug additive.

(iv) Therefore in each year, there is a potential risk of unwanted sequelae of such drug additions with 1·5 million infusion fluids. This risk is increased when multiple drug additives are involved.

Microbiological contamination of intravenous fluids due to drug addition is only one facet of all the possible unwanted sequelae that could result from drug additions (Table 3.3). That there is no good clinical evidence to date in the United Kingdom that drug additions have presented a microbial hazard to the patient would suggest that, although the theoretical hazard may be large (i.e., 1·5 million drug additions to fluids per year), in practice this does not seem to present a clinical problem.

TABLE 3.3   Potential unwanted sequelae of drug addition to intravenous infusion fluids

---

Reduced activity or inactivation of added drug(s)
Altered pharmacokinetic profile of added drug(s)
Incompatibility between drug(s) and fluid or between drugs in fluid
Degradation of infusion fluid
Increased toxicity of added drug (e.g. KCl layering effect)
Bacterial contamination
Pyrogenicity
Increase in particles
Sorption of drugs onto plastics (e.g. vitamin A)
Chemical reactions between plastics container and added drug(s)

3.2.3   In-use contamination rate of intravenous infusions

Work by Woodside and colleagues[17] in the Department of Pharmacy at The Queen's University of Belfast, has provided some data on the contribution of drug addition to microbiological contamination of infusion fluids. All fluid containers were collected from the wards after use and were stored in a refrigerator until sampled. Sampling was done within two hours of collection. Analysis of the residue in 1003 intravenous fluid containers showed a higher incidence of contamination in containers to which drugs had been added (Table 3.4). Bacterial counts per millilitre ranged from eight to uncountable (Table 3.5); highest counts were observed in containers without additives. No contamination was detected in the flexible plastic containers examined, but the number examined was relatively small (3 with additives, 48 without additives).

TABLE 3.4 Analysis of intravenous infusion fluid containers showing contamination (from Woodside et al.[17])

Containers	Total	Number contaminated
With additives	284	19 (6·7%)
Without additives	719	26 (3·6%)
Total	1003	45 (4·5%)

TABLE 3.5 Analysis of colony counts in intravenous fluid samples showing contamination (from Woodside et al.[17])

Count*/ml	Containers with additives	Containers without additives
8–50	18 (40%)	12 (26·7%)
50–100	1 (2·2%)	4 (8·9%)
100–300	—	7 (15·5%)
>300	—	3 (6·7%)

* Streptococci, Staphylococci and Gram-negative rods

TABLE 3.6 In-use contamination rate of intravenous infusion fluids: comparison of data from published work

Authors	Contamination % With additives		Without additives
Miller et al.[18]	8·4–17·7		—
Myers[19]	—	24	—
Hughes[13]	3·3		5·5
Woodside et al.[17]	6·7		3·6
Newman et al.[20]	—		27
Allwood[21] (cites USA data)	—	10	—

In this survey, the most commonly used fluids were 5% dextrose and normal saline, accounting for 85% of the total. No significant difference was detected in the proportion of these fluids showing contamination; in 5% dextrose the incidence of contamination was 3·84% and in normal saline it was 3·55%. Of particular interest was the fact that, of fourteen containers of Rheomacrodex, four showed contamination.

If taken in isolation, the findings of Woodside and his colleagues[17] indicate that addition of drugs to the container contributes significantly to contamination of the fluid. However, other evidence in the literature is not so clear-cut. Comparison of this published evidence (Table 3.6) may not be strictly justifiable since obviously conditions differ from study to study even in such basic procedures as collection and sampling of fluid containers. However, it is the only evidence available and, sparse as it is, such comparison is better than drawing general conclusions from individual sets of data. It may at least act as a guide to indicate what further work should be done. Perusal of Table 3.6 shows clearly that there is no general pattern emerging. Woodside et al.[17] found that additives increased the contamination rate of the fluids; equally clearly Hughes[13] showed the reverse. Myers[19] has reported an overall contamination rate of 24% but did not give any indication whether additives were present. Newman et al.[20] found 27% contamination in fluids without additives and Miller et al.[18] showed 8·4 to 17·7% contamination in fluids containing additives. American data reviewed by Allwood[21] suggests that there is an overall 10% in-use contamination rate for intravenous infusions.

Even if it were assumed that the case was made for drug additives contributing to in-use contamination of intravenous infusions, it is clear that this is not the only source nor even the major source of in-use contamination. It is significant that in the two clear-cut but opposing sets of results of Woodside et al.[17] and Hughes[13], the actual contamination rates experienced were low when compared with the overall in-use contamination rates shown in the limited data available from the other studies. With present data, it must be concluded that incrimination of drug additives as a source of contamination is inconclusive.

3.3 GENERAL CONCLUSIONS

The limited in-use studies on drug additives as a source of microbiological contamination of intravenous infusion fluids do not provide adequate information to draw any firm conclusions. In isolation, individual results could be used to support or reject the incrimination of additives in contamination but taken in toto they are inconclusive.

There is a relative absence of clear-cut, unequivocal clinical reports of drug-additives causing clinical hazard because of microbial contamination. Other clinical hazards of drug additives (e.g., interactions and incompatibilities) have been clearly established[11], so if microbial hazards had occurred then it is reasonable to assume that they would have been recognized and reported. They could, however, be more difficult to detect than say a frank iatrogenic episode. However, since drug addition to infusion fluids is such a common practice, it is unlikely, bearing in mind the volume of fluids used, that the majority of such contamination sequelae would have been missed.

The question whether additives are an additional microbiological hazard of infusion therapy must for the present remain unanswered. Obviously more detailed *in-use* studies would be of value, especially if they followed a uniform protocol and were carried out in different centres. The number of fluid containers sampled must of necessity be large. Also there would be merit in sampling the containers *in situ* before they were removed from the bedside, since the actual dismantling of the giving-set from the container could also be a source of contamination and could bias the *in-use* results. Isolation and identification of contaminating microorganisms (including yeasts and fungi) would provide valuable information on sources of contamination. More clinical study is obviously needed since without some good evidence that additive containing fluids can be a microbiological hazard, the suggested *in-use* studies become largely of academic rather than practical importance. The title of this paper ended with a question mark, which must obviously remain. Drug additives as an additional microbial hazard of infusion therapy care are as yet NOT PROVEN.

References

1. Rosenheim, M. L. (Chairman) (1972). *Interim report on heat sterilized fluids for parenteral administration.* (London: HMSO)
2. Davis, N. and Turco, S. (1971). A study of particulate matter in infusion fluids: Phase 2. *Am. J. Hosp. Pharm.*, **28**, 620
3. Phillips, I. and Eykyn, S. (1972). Contaminated drip fluids. *Br. Med. J.*, **1**, 746
4. Phillips, I., Eykyn, S. and Laker, M. (1972). Outbreak of hospital infection caused by contaminated autoclaved fluids. *Lancet*, **i**, 1258
5. Clothier, C. M. (Chairman) (1972). *Report of the Committee appointed to enquire into the circumstances, including the production, which led to the contaminated infusion fluids in the Devonport Section of Plymouth General Hospital.* (London: HMSO).
6. Meers, P. D., Calder, M. W., Mazhar, M. M. and Lawrie, G. M. (1973). Intravenous infusion of contaminated dextrose solution. The Devonport incident. *Lancet*, **ii**, 1189

7. Editorial (1972). Pharmacy practice. *Pharm. J.*, **208**, 427
8. Rosenheim, M. L. (Chairman) (1973). *Report on the prevention of microbial contamination of medicinal products.* (London: HMSO)
9. D'Arcy, P. F. and Griffin, J. P. (1974). Drug Interactions: 2. By mixing drugs before administration. *Prescribers' J.*, **14**, 38
10. D'Arcy, P. F. and Thompson, K. M. (1974). Drug additives to intravenous infusions: A survey of 10 hospitals in Ulster. *Pharm. J.*, **213**, 172
11. Griffin, J. P. and D'Arcy, P. F. (1975). *A Manual of Adverse Drug Interactions.* pp. 6–13 (Bristol: Wright)
12. Editorial. (1974). Microbiological hazards of intravenous infusions. *Lancet*, **i**, 543
13. Hughes, G. (1973). 24-hour IV service. *Pharm. J.*, **211**, 161
14. Brodlie, P., Henney, C. and Wood, A. J. J. (1974). Problems of administering drugs by continuous infusion. *Br. Med. J.*, **i**, 383
15. Harrison, P. I. and Lowe, I. W. S. (1974). Practical ward study of intravenous additives. *J. Hosp. Pharm.*, **32**, 31
16. Timoney, R. F. and Harte, V. (1974). Personal communication to the author
17. Woodside, W., Woodside, M. E., D'Arcy, P. F. and Patel, R. H. (1975). Intravenous fluids as vehicles of infection. *Pharm. J.*, **215**, 606
18. Miller, W. A., Smith, G. L. and Latiolais, C. J. (1971). A comparative evaluation of compounding costs and contamination rates of intravenous admixture systems. *Drug Intell. Clin. Pharm.*, **5**, 51
19. Myers, J. A. (1972). Millipore infusion filter unit: Interim report of clinical trial. *Pharm. J.*, **208**, 547
20. Newman, M. S., Dempsey, G. and Walker, J. (1975). Microbial and particulate contamination during prolonged use of intravenous infusion sets. *J. Hosp. Pharm.*, **33**, 95
21. Allwood, M. C. (1975). Microbial contamination of sterile fluids in glass containers. *J. Hosp. Pharm.*, **33**, 119

4

Intravenous infusions: The potential for and source of contamination
P. D. Meers

4.1 INTRODUCTION

The microbiological hazards of intravenous therapy comprise but a sub-section of one of the four principal dangers of this kind of treatment. Mechanical, physiological and pharmacological error must be considered in placing the last, that of particulate matter, in perspective. Here we are concerned with the living particle, whose importance was recognized long before that of the inanimate one, which only began to attract general attention a few years ago[1]. Our liquid and gaseous environments contain unimaginably large numbers of microscopic fragments, only a small proportion of which are living. It is salutary to recall that hydraulic and precision engineers have led the way in realizing the importance of con-trolling this kind of contamination. Because microbes represent one kind of particle, attention to the ideas and methods of these engineers is capable of improving the microbiological quality of medical and surgical treatment, quite apart from reducing the mechanical and toxicological dangers to patients of the inanimate fragments to which modern therapy may expose them.

4.2. LIVING PARTICULATE CONTAMINATION AND ITS EFFECTS

The living things which have been found contaminating infusion liquid and the apparatus used to deliver it have ranged from insects to viruses. Pharaoh's ants have been found inside a giving-set[2]. Protozoa and viruses may accompany blood or its products and produce disease in those infused, with malaria and serum (type B) hepatitis being good examples. Crystalloid solutions are most unlikely to transmit such diseases but can act as efficient carriers, and sometimes as amplifiers, of fungi and in particular, of bacteria. The outcome for a patient who is infused with a liquid containing organisms is the resultant of a complex interplay of many factors, which may conveniently be summarized under three headings.

4.2.1 The capacity of the patient to respond to and resist invasion

When primitive single-celled creatures first discovered an advantage in collaboration and began to evolve into multicellular structures, they found it necessary to develop a liquid-filled internal system to bring nutrients to the collaborating cells and take away their waste products. These circu-latory systems would have been ideal havens for the remaining single-celled animals and plants, providing the advantages of evolutionary development without its disadvantages. Battle must have been joined very early in evolutionary history between the smaller creatures trying to get into these systems and the larger ones wanting to keep them out, as even primitive animals with rudimentary blood streams possess biological machinery for attacking and destroying smaller invaders. In man this system consists of multiple, complex interlocking mechanisms, able to deal with a continuous low level of leakage of organisms into the circulation from various surfaces of the body. Intravenous therapy opens an artificial route along which microbes can get into the circulation in varieties and numbers otherwise impossible. The size of microbiological insult delivered in this way that can be overcome by a patient's defences is remarkable, and although illness may weaken these defences and they may be further damaged by some kinds of treatment, some or all of them remain operative. The variability of a patient's response is considerable, and its vigour critical to the outcome, but a consideration of the human factors involved is outside the scope of this Symposium. The result for the patient also depends on the weight of the microbiological challenge with which he is presented. When this is massive, high morbidity and mortality result; when it is very small, there may be no morbidity. Between these extremes patients react differently depending on the size of the challenge and the adequacy of their defensive responses.

4.2.2 The type and number of microbes involved

The microbiological challenge presented to a patient infused with a contaminated solution varies with the type of organism involved and the size and toxicity of its population.

Most classical human pathogens are well adapted to their hosts, and are parasitic to the extent that they are nutritionally demanding, and do not do well outside relatively narrow limits of pH and temperature. Conditions in intravenous fluids rarely satisfy these needs, so that if such organisms get into an infusion, they usually fail to multiply, and may die out quite rapidly. On the other hand saprophytic, free-living organisms are well adapted to survive in poor surroundings, and can multiply using simple nutrients within quite wide limits of pH and temperature. When inoculated into simple intravenous solutions, such organisms may grow into large populations, the final size of which will depend to some extent on the type of fluid involved. The simplest of these in regular use, normal saline, apparently lacks sources of energy, carbon and nitrogen, as well as the essential minerals necessary to the growth of even the least demanding organism, and the addition of dextrose only corrects some of these deficiencies. However, commercially available intravenous fluids contain the essential factors necessary to support the growth of large populations of certain organisms. For instance, a 5% dextrose intravenous solution has been shown to support the growth of over 10^9 *Klebsiella aerogenes* per litre[3]. Such a fluid is turbid when viewed critically with the naked eye, but a less nutritious fluid, or one contaminated with a more demanding organism may develop a smaller but still very large population of bacteria, yet appear perfectly clear. The other variables are the time which elapses between the contamination of a fluid and its injection into a patient, and the temperature at which the fluid is kept. Both these factors are critical, because if properly applied they are capable of converting an innocuously contaminated fluid into one containing a lethal population of microbes.

4.2.3   The amount of toxin formed by microbial growth in a fluid

All growing bacteria produce potentially toxic material. The important toxins in the context of infusion fluids are the pyrogenic endotoxins formed as part of the cell walls of certain Gram-negative organisms. These may be produced by the saprophytic bacteria capable of growing actively in simple intravenous solutions. Endotoxins in an intravenous solution can be detected after the right organisms have grown in it for a few hours, but the amount gradually increases as time passes until the fluid may be so toxic as to be lethal on injection into a patient.

4.3   THE OUTCOME FOR THE PATIENT

The slow development of endotoxin in fluids in which Gram-negative organisms are growing divides the clinical results of an infusion of contaminated fluid into two distinct, though individually heterogeneous, classes. The first of these classes of clinical result follows the infusion of a fluid in the early hours or days after it has been contaminated, when it contains a number of Gram-positive or Gram-negative organisms, but little or no endotoxin. In such a case a patient may suffer no more than transient and perhaps symptomless bacteraemia, or if the organism succeeds in establishing itself in his tissues there follows an illness characterized by the delayed onset of non-specific infective symptoms. This sort of outcome is that which most commonly follows an infusion which introduces bacteria into a patient's circulation. The second class of clinical result follows the infusion of fluid which has been contaminated with toxigenic, usually Gram-negative organisms for a longer time, when although it may contain a diminishing number of living bacteria, it will include an increasing amount of endotoxin. The infusion of such a fluid usually has an instantaneous, dramatic effect, and may be rapidly fatal. This kind of reaction is uncommon, and follows the use of fluids, including whole blood, which were contaminated in their original containers.

4.4 THE ENTRY OF CONTAMINATING ORGANISMS INTO AN INFUSION, AND THEIR ORIGIN

It is convenient to divide the life of an infusion product into three phases covering its manufacture, transport and storage, and use. Each is accompanied by different risks of microbiological contamination and variable outcome when this happens.

4.4.1 Contamination in manufacture

In the circumstances surrounding the compounding and packaging of large volumes of fluid for intravenous use, sterility is not readily achieved. Manufacturers depend on keeping down the multiplication of contaminants and sterilizing the fluid in its final container. The vital checks in this context are the absence of pyrogenicity from the final product, which rules out significant multiplication of Gram-negative organisms in the fluid during manufacture, and the demonstration of low particle counts at various stages in the process, which demonstrates the efficiency of filtration, the cleanliness of the system, and the lack of significant microbial multiplication. Another universal check is to examine the sterility of the finished product. This is a poor test, as it will detect only major failures of sterilization, unless an unacceptably high proportion of the product is used in the process[4].

A manufacturing failure which allows living organisms to survive through processing to reach a finished intravenous product produces a fluid which may appear normal but contain large amounts of endotoxin, and in which the microbes concerned are almost certain to be saprophytes. The proportion of a batch of fluid which may be involved in this way varies upwards from a single container to the largest number which can escape detection by the sterility check being used.

4.4.2 Contamination during transport and storage

This is due to failure of the package. A glass container may develop a hairline crack, or its closure may leak. A plastic pack may be punctured, or a joint or seal fail. Limited leakage may then be followed by the retrograde spread of contaminating organisms into the fluid, followed by resealing of the leak by crystals of solute or by some other change which prevents further tell-tale loss of liquid. Only one or a very small number of containers of any batch of fluid are likely to be involved in this way, but the contamination which results may be heavy, and the fluid toxic.

4.4.3 In-use contamination

This can be divided into special and general cases. The special case is important because two incidents illustrating it, together with the Devonport dextrose affair[3], have led to great changes in the methods of production and use of intravenous solutions, and a general upheaval which has spread to other therapeutic substances. The two incidents were in St Thomas's Hospital in London[5] and a much larger one in America which involved many hospitals using fluids from one commercial source[6]. Both seem to have been due to the penetration of unsterile water into the interstices of bottle closures during manufacture, either due to its use as a spray to cool bottles after autoclaving, or during handling later. The design of the caps of the bottles allowed some of this water to remain in relation to them so that when they were manipulated during the setting up of an infusion, the contaminated water leaked into the intravenous fluid. Inevitably the organisms concerned were of saprophytic species, for nutritionally demanding ones could not have multiplied significantly in the cooling or other contaminating water, or have remained alive in the closure between manufacture and use. In both cases the illnesses which resulted were not such as immediately to throw suspicion on intravenous products, and the identification of their causes and their elimination required the exercise of skill and persistence.

The general case of *in-use* contamination is certainly the most common of the microbiological hazards of intravenous infusions, and it is arguably the least considered. It arises when an infusion and its associated apparatus is sterile when it arrives at a patient's bedside, yet he later develops infusion-related sepsis. In such a case it is clear that the causative microbes can only have got in through one of the gaps or joins in the system. It is instructive to count these. They number a minimum of three in the simplest, providing connection between a plastic bag and the giving-set, between the latter and the cannula or needle, and between this and the patient's vein. The number rises to six if a bottle is used, and readily reaches twelve or more in systems of average complexity to which a drug is added. Most if not all of these joins are made at the bedside, sometimes under the pressure of an emergency. Joins are broken and re-made under even less advantageous conditions when bottles or bags of fluid are changed. The contaminating organisms can only come from the apparatus, from the air, or from the skin of patients or their attendants. The organisms involved in this type of sepsis are predominantly of the kind found on the skin[7], so are mostly Gram-positive, though there is an undercurrent of Gram-negative species, consistent with an increase in the rate of skin colonization by these organisms in hospital patients[8]. This preponderance of organisms originating in the skin coupled with the fact that the outside of apparatus and the air usually have vanishingly small populations of viable bacteria compared even with healthy skin, makes the latter a prime suspect as the source of contaminating organisms. The site of venepuncture attracts attention, for here skin is pierced by a foreign body in circumstances bound to encourage abnormal bacterial multi-plication in direct contact with the system delivering the infusion. In addition, as the skin provides nutritional and other factors which en-courage multiplication of human pathogens, it is tempting to think of this as the place to blame for most local and general sepsis arising from infusions. However, bacteriological examination of the upper and lower surfaces of terminal filters has suggested that contamination comes from above rather than from below[9]. This does not mean that infection at the site of cannulation is not of outstanding importance in infusion related sepsis, but indicates that it does not always spread upwards into the infusion system from its lower end in a way analogous to that well established in urinary drainage apparatus. It follows that some contamina-tion arises as a result of organisms which get in during the assembly and use of intravenous apparatus. The system for allowing air into bottles so that fluid can run out is suspect, particularly when the air filter is removed, but because contamination still happens when plastic bags are substituted for bottles this cannot be the only, or perhaps even an important point of entry.

The only other possibility is that contamination gets in during the making of joins in the delivery system. Although the hands of a person doing this carry a large bacterial population, it is assumed that direct contact between hands and critical parts of the apparatus are too rare to produce the observed rates of contamination. However the skin is con-stantly shedding squames some of which carry bacteria as can be shown quite readily by the use of a slit-sampler. People gently rubbing their hands together 15 cm above the slit of a sampler (Figure 4.1) can be shown on average to contribute three extra bacteria-carrying particles each 15 seconds to the count on the collecting plate. It is known that washing

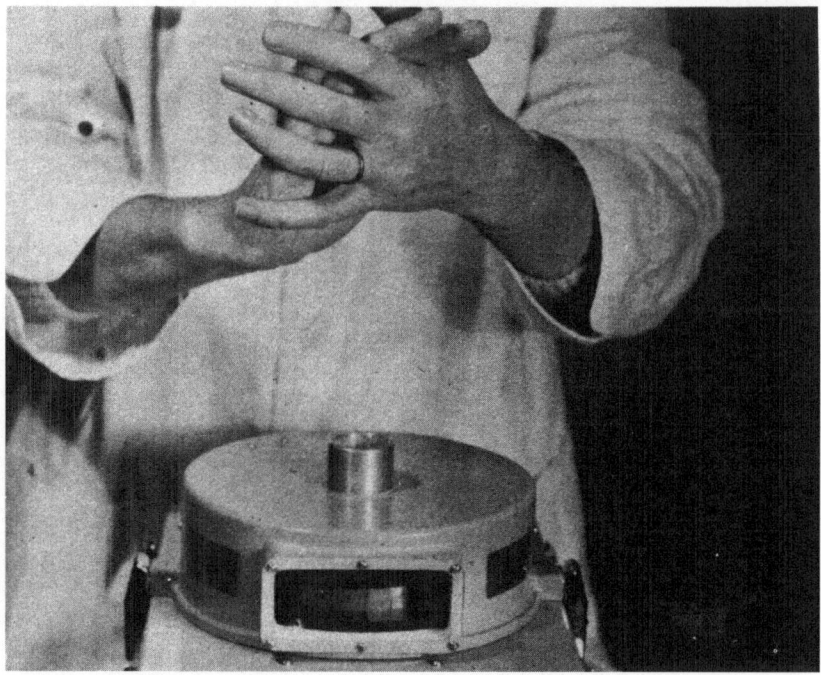

Figure 4.1   A slit sampler being used to collect skin-squames released from hands by gentle rubbing

increases the release of such particles from the body[10], and that this is also true of the hands is borne out by repeating the slit sampler experiment immediately after washing them with toilet soap and drying them on a paper towel. This procedure at least doubles the release of potentially infective particles, and in 50% of people it increases it ten-fold or more (Table 4.1). Even more striking is the fact that some people become amazingly active disseminators of these particles after washing their hands, shedding many hundreds of them in a 15 second period (Figure 4.2). In any one individual the effect is reproducible quantitatively on successive days (Table 4.2). It is clear that the air immediately round each of the multiple sites handled during the setting up of an infusion contains more, and sometimes very many more organisms than are present in the air in general. A contaminated particle, perhaps attracted by static electricity, which adheres to part of a join which is subsequently in direct contact with the infusion fluid contaminates the latter from the outset. If the particle is trapped in the join not in direct contact with the fluid, it may get in later

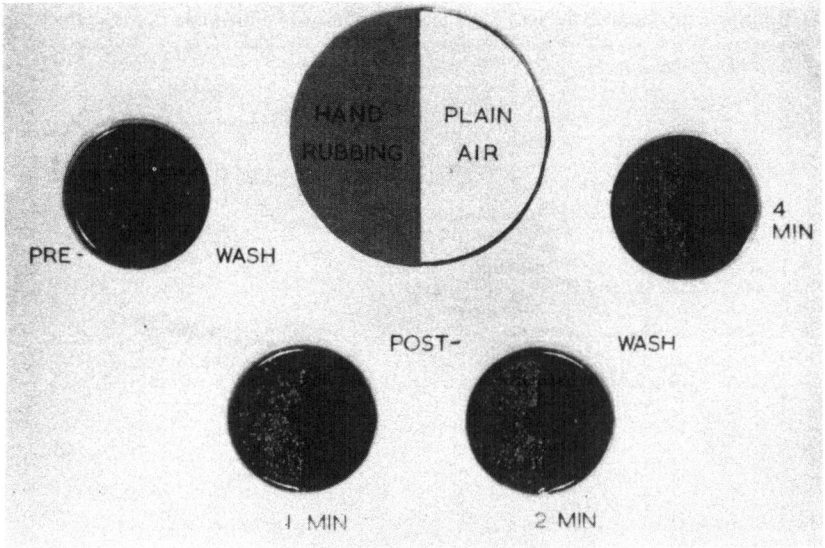

Figure 4.2 Petri-dishes of blood-agar, initially exposed in a slit sampler, after incubation for 24 hours at 37 °C. In each case the right-hand ('plain air') half of the plate bears the growth resulting from a 15 second, 7·5 l, air sample; while the left-hand ('hand rubbing') half results from an exposure for the same time, but made as described in Figure 4.1. The four plates are the result of several exposures from the hands of the same person, before they were washed ('pre-wash'), and at the time intervals shown after washing them, using warm running water and toilet soap and drying them with paper towels as described in the footnote to Table 4.1. The person concerned was individual 3 in Table 4.2

due to movements of the tubing, or with greater certainty when a join is broken and remade. This takes place principally at the upper end, when second or subsequent containers of fluid are given through the same delivery apparatus, though it may also happen elsewhere. This delayed transfer can be demonstrated experimentally by applying a small amount of a radioisotope to the outside of a join between a container of fluid and a giving-set, and examining the effluent from the lower end for radioactivity. In such an experiment, using ^{125}I-labelled human serum albumen, no radioactivity was detected in the effluent from the first bags in eight identical systems, though it was detected in the effluent of three of the eight after the first change of bag, in seven of the eight after two changes, and in all eight after the third. Fortunately, many of the organisms concerned will be of nutritionally demanding Gram-positive species so will

TABLE 4.1 Counts of colony-forming units released from the hands of 20 medical and para-medical personnel by gentle rubbing immediately before and after washing*

Individual No.	Colony-forming units A_1	B	A_2	C
1	3	6	2	33
2	1	9	0	54
3	2	9	13	> 500
4	3	3	1	27
5	5	16	9	21
6	3	10	6	7
7	2	8	6	144
8	8	8	4	29
9	1	2	4	67
10	5	9	9	131
11	6	6	6	49
12	3	6	3	9
13	4	4	5	117
14	2	6	3	13
15	5	5	4	57
16	0	1	4	7
17	2	6	1	19
18	3	2	3	11
19	0	7	1	9
20	0	3	1	10

* The counts were made with a Casella slit-sampler, impinging 15 litres of air in 30 seconds on to a Petri-dish of horse-blood agar, the first 15 seconds (180°) sampling air alone (columns A_1 and A_2) and the second 15 seconds (180°) sampling air with the hands being rubbed together 15 cm above the slit before (column B) and after (column C) washing the hands with running water and toilet soap, and drying them on a paper towel. The paper towels were shown not to contribute to the counts recorded.

TABLE 4.2 Counts recorded as in Table 4.1 by 3 individuals on 5 different days, to demonstate reproducibility of results

Individual No. 2				Individual No. 3				Individual No. 10			
A_1	B	A_2	C	A_1	B	A_2	C	A_1	B	A_2	C
1	9	0	54	2	9	13	> 500	5	9	9	131
0	2	4	36	0	3	12	> 500	4	8	5	60
1	3	1	135	2	5	3	250	5	10	9	64
2	5	2	65	3	4	6	240	8	20	9	95
2	10	1	161	3	22	11	300	2	3	15	70

not multiply in the fluid in the giving-set to any extent (unless the system is being used for infusing whole blood or some other unusually nutritive solution), though contamination with less nutritionally demanding organisms will be followed by active multiplication at this site. On reaching the patient however, any fibrin deposit or larger clot round the needle or cannula provide the nutrients and conditions suitable for the multiplication of most organisms, including the more fastidious ones.

This review of the potential for and sources of the microbiological contamination of intravenous fluids underlines the vital importance to the patient of the protective mechanisms which clear organisms from his blood, as there can be very few infusions which do not expose him to at least some of them. Modern giving-sets are essentially sophisticated copies in plastic of the early glass and rubber apparatus used for transfusing blood. It is interesting to speculate on the design which might emerge if a modern team were asked to produce a system for delivering fluid intravenously if this were to be attempted for the first time today.

References

1. Garvan, J. H. and Gunner, B. W. (1964). The harmful effects of particles in intravenous fluids. *Med. J. Aust.*, **2**, 1
2. Beatson, S. H. (1973). Pharaoh's ants enter giving-sets. *Lancet*, **i**, 606
3. Meers, P. D., Calder, M. W., Mazhar, M. M. and Lawrie, G. M. (1973). Intravenous infusion of contaminated dextrose solution. *Lancet*, **ii**, 1189
4. Kelsey, J. C. (1972). The myth of surgical sterility. *Lancet*, **ii**, 1301
5. Phillips, I., Eykyn, S. and Laker, M. (1972). Outbreak of hospital infection caused by contaminated autoclaved fluids. *Lancet*, **i**, 1258
6. Mackel, D. C., Maki, D. G., Anderson, R. L., Rhame, F. S. and Bennett, J. V. (1975). Nationwide epidemic of septicaemia caused by contaminated intravenous products: mechanisms of intrinsic contamination. *J. Clin. Microbiol.*, **2**, 486
7. Maki, D. G., Goldman, D. A. and Rhame, F. S. (1973). Infection control in intravenous therapy. *Ann. Intern. Med.*, **79**, 867
8. Pollack, M., Charache, P., Nieman, R. E., Jett, M. P., Reinhardt, J. A. and Hardy, P. H. (1972). Factors influencing colonisation and antibiotic-resistance patterns of Gram-negative bacteria in hospital patients. *Lancet*, **ii**, 668
9. Wilmore, D. W. and Dudrick, S. J. (1969). An in-line filter for intravenous solutions. *Arch. Surg.*, **99**, 462
10. Speers, R., Bernard, H., O'Grady, F. and Shooter, R. A. (1965). Increased dispersal of skin bacteria into the air after showerbaths. *Lancet*, **i**, 478

DISCUSSION

Sources, control and detection of contamination
Panel: I. Phillips (in the chair),
P. F. D'Arcy, R. Hambleton,
D. G. Maki and P. D. Meers

1 THE STERLIZATION PROCESS

Dr J. B. KAY (London): I should like to discuss the microbiological hazards in the manufacture of the infusion product itself in the light of Dr Maki's discourse on product-testing. Dr Hambleton has identified various stages in the processing of a packaged product that could present risk, and divided them into pre- and post-sterilization.

Looking at how the microbiological hazards of processing such products can be reduced to a minimum, it is clear that sterilization itself is a physical process involving engineering, and not microbiology, and the Department of Health in the United Kingdom will not recommend the use of microbiological systems either for controlling the process or for indicating that the process has been achieved and would regard it as a time- and temperature-measuring exercise which is a combination of engineering and physics. It is not regarded as a microbiological monitoring exercise.

The Department recommends the purchase of sterilizers conforming to a British Standard, BS 3970 as in departmental publication CS 21. They should be installed using the guidance in HTM 10, and maintained using Maintenance Guides 12 and 13. If all that is done correctly then clearly the product will be sterile. The retrospective testing of the 'Devonport Incident' fluids was totally unnecessary; one had only to look at the records for the batch that caused infection.

Dr MAKI (Madison, Wisconsin): What a familiar bit of 'bureaucratese'. It seems to be common to our two countries. I concur it *is* extremely important to assess the efficacy of the sterilization process by physico-chemical methods. However, at least two major epidemics of infusion-related sepsis traced to intrinsic contamination were not due to failure of the sterilization process, but rather occurred because something un-predictable happened *after* the sterilization process[*],[†]. In such a circum-stance one can examine as many autoclave temperature charts as one wants to, and test biological indicators, till the cows come home, and one will not detect that kind of contamination.

I am not suggesting that product sterility testing is infallible, and will automatically pick up every problem. Contamination can be of such a low level that a practical programme might not pick it up. But it may be possible to devise meaningful programmes that can pick up at least the level of contamination that we have seen in two US nationwide outbreaks (i.e., 6 units per thousand)[*],[†].

[*] See Chapter 2, reference 7
[†] See Chapter 2, reference 31

Professor PHILLIPS (London): Dr Maki seems to be in agreement with Dr Kay.

Dr KAY: Dr Maki is one jump ahead!

Dr MAKI: I do not propose to replace physico-chemical monitoring of the actual sterilizing process. I rather want to *complement* it with something that can detect the unpredictable sequence of events leading to intrinsic contamination as has occurred.

Dr KAY: The design of the product has to be such that it is fit for its intended use. If, in the design of the container physical parameters (for instance, acceptable variations in component size) are laid down, and the manner of manufacture of the components is properly monitored, and the components are tested with proper systems, and the people who use the components are educated, for example to screw bottles down to a fixed torque, the system works. Clearly if the component system was not designed for accelerated cooling, then no one but a fool would use it for that purpose. If the product is ensheathed in microbes such that they enter the product when somebody pierces it, then that is an abuse of the container system which should be avoided by the use of common sense and the allocation of funds to promote commonsense, rather than the funding of microbiological screening.

Dr HAMBLETON (Manchester): To some extent Dr Kay and I are on the same side. One should be able to design a suitable system. I am rather concerned that many systems that are in use have not been evaluated under appropriate conditions. The immmediate problem is to sort out the relevant conditions.

The comments on sterilizers are self-evident. One can design and operate sterilizers correctly, but one should not take that in isolation. Whatever is put into a sterilizer is sterile at the end of the cycle, and so long as it is left in the sterilizer, presumably it will remain so. The trouble is that it must be taken out and used, which is really where many of the problems begin.

2 ENDOTOXIN

UNIDENTIFIED: Dr Maki mentioned the *Limulus* test. I am not sure that it is as good as the official tests. Does it pick up Gram-positive as well as Gram-negative organisms?

Dr MAKI: The test is technically demanding. It is fraught with a fair amount of false positivity, and it is not sufficiently sensitive to pick up levels of contamination with 100 organisms per ml or less. It is also positive with polynucleotides and other non-endotoxic substances*.

Professor D'ARCY (Belfast): With all due respect, I would far sooner see a temperature rise in a rabbit than see a result of a *Limulus* test.

Professor PHILLIPS: How does Dr Meers do his investigations for endotoxin?

Dr MEERS (Plymouth): We used the *Limulus* test, and we did it in a spectrophotometer.

Dr P. J. BRADLEY (Birmingham): Dr Meers showed a slide which related the development of endotoxins in contaminated solutions stored for about a year. If they reach such levels (3 g per litre) I find it most disquieting. Perhaps pharmacists should be looking at old stocks and re-examining them for quality control in that aspect. If we were to consider doing this for manufactured solutions, how should we set about it?

Dr MEERS: I am sure that there is no need to be bothered about it. Such a load of endotoxin will only occur in rather special cases where an organism has got in in the first place and has been allowed to grow for that length of time. To go round testing every conceivable container for the presence of endotoxins would be totally non-cost effective.

The purpose of the slide was to demonstrate what happened to the patients in Devonport who were infused with the fluid, and why they died so quickly. They died of endotoxic shock.

Dr BRADLEY: I was thinking about stocks that may be stored for up to three years.

Dr MEERS: I cannot conceive of any reason for doing it. It is like testing tins of corned beef for Salmonellae. It is a waste of time.

Dr J. G. WALLACE (Lincoln): Are 10^7 organisms as visible inside a double-wrapped plastic bag as they are in a nice clean bottle?

Dr MEERS: I was speaking of bottles, and that was my experience. The opacity was difficult to see, and it was not seen by some of the nursing staff who were reasonable intelligent folk, who might have been expected to see it had it been obvious. It only became obvious when a number of bottles had been assembled and were looked at critically. It would probably have been invisible inside a Viaflex bag, and quite invisible in a 'Polyfusor'.

* See Chapter 2, reference 75

3 ADDITIVES

Dr MAKI: It is very interesting that Professor D'Arcy's non-additive group had a higher mean concentration of microorganisms than the additive group. I would suggest that a larger proportion of the non-additive group had 'keep-open' infusions. As such, their sets probably infused continuously for longer periods than the additive group. Taking into account that introduced microorganisms require up to 12–24 hours to initiate growth*, this might explain in part the differences found.

Professor D'ARCY: Dr Maki is probably absolutely right. There are so many different things that have to be followed: running time, manipulation, etc. . . . There is a danger of taking just one set of observations and drawing a lot of conclusions from it.

Professor PHILLIPS: I know of a case to illustrate just that. Superficially the problem was due to the addition of Pitocin to a drip—an additive problem. Actually the infusion had been put up, turned off for twelve hours, and then started again, and it was probably not an additive problem at all, but one of over-long infusion.

Dr J. H. S. FOSTER (London): To pick up the point about the differential levels of contamination with the additive, would not a possible explanation be that it is the nature of the additive? Antibiotics were listed as a significant number of additives, and in addition such substances as potassium chloride might also have growth-suppressive action.

   Secondly, has Professor D'Arcy any information regarding the conditions under which those additives were made? If those additions were made in the open ward, then it is very likely that contamination could arise. If, on the other hand, they were made with even non-sterile gloves under a laminar flow hood, that would surely produce a very much lower level of contamination when additives are added.

Professor D'ARCY: They were all done in the ward situation, without the benefit of laminar flow. In that respect they are comparable. We were most anxious to take a typical ward situation, and not so much an artificial one where we monitored how the addition was made. As to which additives they were, I regret that that was not recorded. I do take the questioner's point. Some of the additives could have been antibiotics.

Professor PHILLIPS: The only problems that I have seen associated with additives have been either with heparin or Pitocin drips, in use for pro-

* See Chapter 2, reference 15

longed periods which takes me back to an earlier point. Is it really the additives at all?

Professor D'ARCY: There were two recent cases in the City Hospital, Belfast, where two patients showed a dramatic cyclic rise in temperature with heparin and sodium chloride. We did a pyrogen test on the batches of the sodium chloride, and on the sodium chloride with the same amount of heparin added. There was no pyrogenicity at all. I do not know what caused it, but it was not the fluid, and it was not the additive. It is the sort of problem we face.

Dr G. AYLIFFE (Birmingham): Professor D'Arcy has not really demonstrated in his studies the necessity for a laminar air cabinet.

Professor D'ARCY: I am a great believer in belt and braces. I should prefer to have a laminar flow in a ward situation than to do it in a ward situation without a laminar flow. It is an added safeguard.

Dr AYLIFFE: I do not entirely accept that. The evidence does not show it.

Dr HAMBLETON: One would need to be very careful about installing laminar flow units haphazardly here and there. When a laminar flow unit is turned off, dust collects, and then when it is turned on, there is a lovely dust cloud, and unless people are aware of this problem, and take steps to see that it does not happen, the whole object of using a laminar flow cabinet might be defeated.

Professor D'ARCY: Obviously that is not what was intended. I merely think that a laminar flow cabinet is better than no laminar flow cabinet.

Mr E. R. TALLETT (Burnley): The job is a job for the pharmacist. There are many other important things besides bacterial contamination. If the job is handed over to a pharmacist, and he is given good conditions, it will be well done.

Professor D'ARCY: I would agree. However, in three years of negotiations with the Area Boards, we are no nearer to getting the conditions, or the pharmacists, or the salary structure, or the 24-hour service. Our nursing colleagues are still having to do it, and I cannot see any light at the end of that tunnel.

In Belfast at the moment we are just starting a 24-hour service in one of our hospitals as an experiment. We hope that it will continue, but whether it does will largely depend on whether we can get the pharmacy staff and the establishment to run it.

I entirely agree with Mr Tallett, but he and I are preaching in a wilderness.

Mr TALLETT: But let us not preach laminar flow on the wards. The place for a laminar flow screen is in the pharmacy, where in addition to that minor problem of contamination, all the other problems can be dealt with by competent personnel.

Professor D'ARCY: I do agree, but who will do it after 5 o'clock on Friday night?

Mr TALLET: Pharmacists in Burnley!

Professor D'ARCY: That must be the only place at the moment.

Dr MAKI: The pharmacists at the University of Wisconsin compound intravenous admixtures 24 hours a day. The system works exceedingly well, and I would be loath to go back to the old system.

Mr L. A. GOLDBERG (Manchester): 100% of all peritoneal dialysis containers have additions made to them, and there is an incidence of somewhere between 15 and 20% peritonitis as a result of the procedure. Surely the same criteria must be adopted for peritoneal dialysis solutions, or else industry must be persuaded to add drugs like heparin to the solutions as is done with potassium chloride.

Professor D'ARCY: We would like to do a similar study on dialysis solutions. Until one has done one of these studies, one does not realize what time and trouble it takes—just to have enough students to run backwards and forwards from the wards. If anybody has the time and the inclination to do it, the evidence that they will get will be useful, but it needs a lot more information.

Mr GOLDBERG: In the ward, it is fairly common for staff to prepare the first 12 or 24 litres of peritoneal dialysis solution, by making the necessary additions then putting the fluid into a suitable incubator at body temperature for 12–18 hours; and then they wonder why peritonitis ensues.

4 IN-USE CONTAMINATION

Mr R. PURKISS (Cambridge): We ran an in-use survey at Addenbrookes Hospital, taking samples of infusion fluids and giving-sets, all of which had 100 ml or more of infusion left. None of the giving-sets had been up for more than 24 hours, and the infusion fluids had been up for a range of times. The infusion fluids were both in bottles that had been manufactured in the hospital and bags which had been brought in. In 60 samples taken over a period of two months, five of them having had a single additive, we found no contamination at all. We used the membrane filtration method, and we incubated the membranes in three different media and found no contamination.

Dr MAKI: That does not surprise me. The rate of contamination in various hospitals has ranged from $0·9\%$ in a hospital sampling over a thousand systems over a given period of time to as high as 9%. Some of the earlier studies that found 20 or 30% were unrepresentative; some of them took place during outbreaks due to intrinsically contaminated products. However if in-use contamination of over 5% occurs and total-volume sampling has been employed, I should wonder if the hospital had an ongoing problem, or if their sampling procedure was introducing contamination.

Mr N. GEE (Burnley): Dr Maki mentioned the use of in-line filters to reduce contamination to the patient. However they present a danger. There is the possibility of the in-line filter puncturing, and the patient getting a bolus injection of the bacteria that may have settled on the filter.

Dr MAKI: A manufacturer of filters could retort to that by stating that without the filter the bacteria would get in anyhow. I am not too concerned about a filter malfunctioning. I am more concerned that if a filter plugs, then a predictable sequence of events occurs. The nurse goes to the bed-side and starts to manipulate the system; she looks at the cannula, may irrigate it a few times before she finally comes to the realization that the filter is responsible. My fear is that these added manipulations increase considerably the risk of contamination. There are uncontrolled data to suggest that this hazard of filters is read and not properly appreciated[5].

Filters are of theoretical value, but they have not been proven useful in preventing disease (except possibly phlebitis[6]) in any clinical trials of which I am aware.

Dr J. M. T. HAMILTON-MILLER (Royal Free Hospital): Has Dr Maki ever found anaerobic organisms in any fluids? Some of them fix CO_2 and nitrogen, and I should imagine that after autoclaving there would be an anaerobic system.

* See Chapter 7, reference 113
† See Chapter 7, reference 117

Dr MAKI: We have no data on anaerobic organisms. The media that we use in our studies will not support the growth of anaerobes. Studies that others have done, using thioglycolate as a growth media, have shown anaerobic diphtheroids; but I am unaware of any other anerobic species than that which has been received from fluids.

On empirical grounds I would be dubious that anaerobes play any important role in infections related to contaminated fluids, but I confess that unless somebody looks at it rigorously, it would be hard to make this statement categorically.

Mr J. A. MYERS (Edinburgh): In how many cases, apart from the four major cases Dr Maki mentioned, have bacteria in the bottle caused infection in the patient?

Dr MAKI: I shall be addressing that tomorrow. It is a very difficult question which I have thought about for a long time. What is the significance of *infection* caused by extrinsic contamination? It appears to be quite low.

Mr MYERS: Quite often if it is suggested to a doctor that the set be changed every 24 hours, he will say that he had considerable difficulty in finding a suitable vein, and he will not touch it, even though it becomes infected, until the vein becomes grossly damaged.

Dr MAKI: I did not say that it was necessary to change a cannula every 24 hours. I am a clinician and keenly realize that it is not practical to charge cannulae every 24 hours. One might like to do it but it is not realistic. I was referring to changing the *administration set*. It is recommendable to change the entire delivery apparatus (all bottles and giving-sets) down to the cannula every 24–48 hours and certainly every time the cannula is replaced.

Dr R. Y. CARTRIGHT (Guildford): First, a comment. A number of the speakers have mentioned the problem of design, and that it is important to consult the user when apparatus is designed. So often the manufacturers will talk to the medical staff, but they fail to realize that the most important user in intravenous therapy is the junior nurse, operating at three o'clock in the morning, in a poorly-lit ward, and probably with somebody calling from the other end of the ward. The system has to be capable of coping with that situation.

Secondly, does Dr Meers now instruct his medical nursing staff not to wash their hands before giving intravenous fluids?

Dr MEERS: I confess to being very surprised by the results that I showed.

I produced the results during March 1976 for the purposes of this Symposium, and I have not yet told many people about it. The horror which will strike at the breasts of our nursing colleagues if we do say that will pass belief! I mentioned it because it seemed worth bringing out as something which people can try for themselves.

Professor PHILLIPS: Has it been shown that organisms on skin scales, in the form of dandruff, stick to the cannula during the actual manipulation?

Dr MEERS: No, but I am sure that it all hangs together.

Dr G. AYLIFFE (Birmingham): A comment on hand washing. It removes most of the transient organisms, including the Gram-negative bacilli.

I wonder whether the other organisms which are left have any clinical relevance in this situation.

Dr MEERS: They are mostly *Staphylococcus epidermidis*, or related organisms. The published figures for in-use contamination of intravenous fluids, give *Staphylococcus epidermidis* as the commonest contaminant. This *may* be regarded as a non-pathogen, but undoubtedly is the commonest organism and I am suggesting that hands are the source of it. I do not know if it is important.

5 STERILITY TESTING

Mr G. SYKES (London): I should like to discuss methods of sterility testing. Filtration may be inferior in some respects to adding a concentrated medium, but there are problems with adding concentrated medium. One is limited to testing solutions which are virtually isotonic, and medium cannot be added to a 20% dextrose concentration because that medium is inhibitory to microbial growth. There is also a restriction in terms of testing bags of fluid in that in the first place there is no space in a properly filled bag to put in the medium, and in the second place, if there were, there would not be any airspace to provide oxygen for the growth of the obligate aerobes.

Dr MAKI: In my laboratory we have used the hyperconcentrated broth method with bag containers, in a laminar flow hood, and it works well. We put in about 25–50 ml of ten-fold concentrated medium per 1000 ml. We have not found a need to add air. We are satisfied that the technique has minimal sampling error. We have also shown that we could innoculate a very small number of organisms (estimated at about 10 organisms) into the bag, and it would rapidly turn turbid, within 24 hours. With gas-forming organisms care should be taken as the bag can burst if not correctly vented.

The hyperconcentrated method can work with the bag. It takes some modification but can be done with a minimum of sampling error, and it is very simple.

Mr SYKES: On another point, the method of incubation of membranes, if I remember rightly they are incubated at 35–37 °C for 48 hours, and then five days at room temperature. That is the wrong way around. Organisms that will grow at room temperature may easily be killed if they are incubated for a prolonged period, i.e. 24–48 hours, at 37 °C. The right way round for incubation if it is to be done in this dual manner is to incubate at room temperature for a few days, and then put it up to 37 °C.

Dr MAKI: I don't know and doubt if anyone can tacitly say which is the best sequence. Maybe if an organism can grow at 37 °C, it is more likely to be pathogenic and to cause problems to a patient.

Coming back to the basic philosophy, I have not stated that the hyperconcentrated broth is the best way to sample fluid. But, it does seem to be more sensitive than the membrane filtration technique. The USA method currently in use (membrane filtration) may be inadequate in other respects. If we were to go back in time, and look at the data in the USA Abbott incident, we would note a striking increase in their quality control positives in the year of their epidemic*. Yet nothing was done with that data. It may or may not have been related to the epidemic. The recovered organisms were unidentified. But the epidemic pointed to inadequacies in the quality control system. If they had identified the organisms, and had found that there was an *Enterobacter agglomerans*, a then unusual organism, even in only one unit five or six months earlier—we knew that there were patients in American hospitals getting septicaemia with this rare pathogen—hundreds of cases of septicaemia might have been prevented.

What I am asking is for a critical re-examination of our current quality control sampling programmes, including methods of sampling and microbiological identification, collation of data and reporting of results to a central monitoring agency.

Mr SYKES: We have been talking about Utopia, or Shangri-La, or some place of that nature. We are not there yet, nor are we likely to be for some while.

* See Chapter 2, reference 7

There is no doubt that the primary control must be with the sterilization process, but we have not yet reached a stage at which we can say that we can dispense with the final tests. It ought to be the aim of any quality controller in any branch of pharmaceutical manufacture, and it will be in the end, but in the meantime, we shall have to stick to a form of testing, particularly where there is no control on the possible breakdown of a closure or of some other system after sterilization.

Testing will not pick out the odd 1 or 2% of those things that may happen, but cumulative testing will give us more assurance. I do not rely on, or place any credence in, the single test on a single batch. It is the cumulative evidence which is important, and that is what we should aim for, and ultimately get rid of the tests for sterility.

Mr E. MITCHELL (London): The major problem seems to be stopping people from dying because they have been given very large numbers of microbes in transfused fluid. Perhaps we, as microbiologists, working in our cottage industry, should be thinking more of the use of electronic devices to detect large numbers of microbes as the final screen, rather than the culture plate and the loop.

Dr MEERS: Particle counting is a way of counting small things, and some of these things are likely to be living. The pharmacopeias of most advanced countries include criteria for the number of particles allowed in infusion fluids, but it is interesting to note that the EEC Pharmacopeia—to which we in the UK will have to conform shortly—has no criteria for such particles at present.

Dr MAKI: The infusion of massive numbers of organisms leading to the catastrophic endotoxic shock syndrome is fortunately rare, and is almost exclusively confined to one of two circumstances. First, where there has been a breakdown in manufacturing, sterility control and *fluid* (not the closure) becomes contaminated by organisms that subsequently multiply to very high concentrations. Secondly, there is the rare instance of a crack in a bottle and a similar sequence of events. Up to now I have been emphasizing post-autoclave intrinsic contamination. Most of the item those organisms that get into the fluid when it is set up for use (extrinsic contamination) fail to propagate to levels where they can cause significant illness. Emphasis on detection of contamination in the manufacturing part of the entire sequence should cut down on such catastrophes more than electronic surveillance at the bedside.

Dr MITCHELL: That would be lovely in the ideal world where every bottle goes through the autoclave, and no bottle dodges quality control.

But for the bad situation, where the bottle is neither sterilized, nor quality controlled, and yet finds its way to the bedside looking like any other bottle, some kind of final check is needed. If one can look for particles, at that stage, with more sophisticated equipment, it may be cheaper than microbiology.

Dr MAKI: If it can be made easily, and it can be cheap (ideally less than £1 per unit), and it can fit into the palm of the hand, and the infusion line could be run through it, then none of us would disagree.

Professor PHILLIPS: We note that for future action.

Dr R. Y. CARTRIGHT: We have talked about testing just before the product is given to the patient. If it is to be tested within a hospital, should it be tested when it arrives in the hospital, when it has been in the pharmacy store for so long, or just before it is given to the patient?

The biggest practical problem is that in most hospitals there are not the people, or the necessary apparatus, to do the testing, so we are discussing something that is purely theoretical for the vast majority. Surely what is most important is that we have a system whereby anybody who suspects trouble associated with infusion fluids gets in touch with the right people who can take the right action immediately, and that must apply at any time of the day or the night on any day of the year. That is the practical approach to detection for contamination. It is not ideal, but in practice it is probably the best that can be done.

Dr MAKI: I hope that that was the thrust of my paper. Detection of clinical illness is the final screen, and an extremely important one in detecting a major problem. But I believe back in the manufacturing plant we can also do something of preventive value.

I cannot agree more fully that the cost benefit of sampling programmes in the hospital is not proven. As I stated in my paper I know of no on-going sampling programmes in the United States that have detected clinical infections caused by contaminated fluid although a number of hospitals have quite sophisticated programmes. These hospitals however might conceivably detect a major problem in the future.

Mr SYKES: The situation is different in the UK. In the USA, intra-venous fluid is not made in the hospitals, whereas here 50% of them are made in the hospitals, and therefore there needs to be some system of testing, as there is for industry.

Testing for microbial contamination, or for sterility, is not a job to be done by anybody at any time. It should not be done in every hospital.

Every region needs only one, or possibly two, specialist labs which can do this kind of work. Unless that kind of confined control is used, one is testing the tests and not the product.

Professor PHILLIPS: We all agree on that. Many of us would be relieved if such facilities existed.

SECTION TWO

Clinical Problems
Chairman:
Professor P. F. D'Arcy

5

Clinical syndromes
A. M. Geddes

5.1 INTRODUCTION

There are considerable differences, in various parts of the world, in the incidence of infection associated with intravenous infusion. For example, the problem appears to be much less common in Britain than in the USA and Canada. This is probably associated with regional differences in the preferred route of administration of drugs. Intravenous therapy, both for the correction of imbalance and for the administration of drugs, is much less often undertaken in Britain than in the USA. This is not a criticism. It is in part due to the fact that we have probably been slower in setting up intensive care units which regularly use the intravenous route for investigation and therapy, often unnecessarily.

The East Birmingham Hospital is a large district general hospital of approximately a thousand beds, with most clinical disciplines represented. What follows relates to our own experience of infections associated with intravenous infusions.

5.2 INTRINSIC CONTAMINATION

Our experience with intrinsic contamination of intravenous infusion fluid is extremely limited, as it probably is in most other British hospitals. We have in fact recognized only one episode during the past ten years. The fluid on that occasion was blood contained in one of the early plastic infusion packs. The patient was recovering after a Caesarian section and was given a blood transfusion. When half of the contents of the pack had been infused she suddenly collapsed. A mismatched transfusion was immediately thought of but no-one considered septicaemia: her state of shock became irreversible and she died. Blood collected at post-mortem and from the infusion pack yielded a profuse growth of a *Klebsiella* species.

In stating that this kind of episode is rare, I would point out that in the average general hospital in the UK only about 30% of patients who die have post-mortem examinations, and it is therefore impossible to state categorically that we have only seen one in 10 years. We have only *identified* one in 10 years, and I suspect that patients die from microbiological hazards of infusion therapy which go unrecognized, death being attributed to pulmonary embolism or to myocardial infarction, which can so easily mimic septic shock, particularly in the elderly. Even with a post-mortem the diagnosis may be missed, unless the pathologist is considering septicaemia, and cultures blood and body fluids to make the diagnosis. The terminal stages of septic shock may well mimic myocardial infarction because myocarditis is one of the pathological processes.

Before leaving the fluid itself, I should like to make a plea against unnecessary parenteral nutrition. Patients are given parenteral nutrition, with amino acid and alcohol-containing fluids, often without due thought being given to the potential hazards, and, on a number of occasions I have seen so-called 'hyperalimentation' being prescribed during the course of a chronic illness, when it was unnecessary; a young resident had just read about the solution and considered that this was the thing to do for his patient. I would counsel pharmacists, especially, that they should educate young doctors and remind them when they order parenteral nutrition of the potential hazards associated with this form of therapy.

5.3 CARE OF THE INFUSION

Too often infusions are not set up as a sterile procedure. One of the problems that has always worried me, although hopefully it will now change, is the infusion containers which have a spout on the end which has to be cut off with a pair of scissors. Not infrequently I see nurses reaching into their pockets, taking out a pair of scissors, and cutting off that snout with them! I understand that the containers have recently been changed, and that there should be some improvement in the snout which is now to be capped.

Ideally, the drip set should be changed every 24 hours and this is not difficult. In addition, whenever blood has been given through a drip set, the set should probably be changed. One can go around the wards and see a patient who has had a blood transfusion and who is now being given saline or glucose through the same apparatus, and observe the blood clogging up the filters. Surely blood trapped in a filter being washed by glucose must be an excellent culture medium.

5.4 ADDITIVES

Once the infusion has been set up, a potentially dangerous procedure is the addition of drugs to the infusion bottle. Infection traced to this practice is, however, surprisingly uncommon, even following grossly erroneous procedures. I can give a recent example. Cotrimoxazole for infusion is given as two ampoules added to 200 ml of sodium chloride, and I saw a nurse reading the instructions, unscrewing the top of a sodium chloride bottle, decanting 300 ml, setting it down, going off to answer the phone, coming back, and then adding the two ampoules, as if she was working in the kitchen—a little of this, a little of that—screwing it on again and setting it up.

There are remarkably few instances when additives *are* required. Antibiotics are my own interest, and the addition of antibiotics to infusion fluids is very, very seldom necessary. If they must be given by the intravenous route, then they should be injected by bolus into the drip set or a cannula, and not added to infusion fluid.

I know that the subject has already been discussed, but it is important to stress that if drugs are to be added to infusion fluids, the procedure must be performed aseptically, preferably in the pharmacy, and, ideally, a 24-hour additive service provided by the pharmacy would obviate the need for the nurses to do it in the ward. I should certainly like to see such a service for that and also other reasons.

5.5   DRIP SITE INFECTION

In the UK and in our experience, drip site infection is probably the most potent cause of infection associated with infusion therapy. In the last 6 months within our own hospital we have had three septicaemias, two of them fatal, originating in an infected drip site. The organisms were *Staphylococcus aureus*, *Serratia marcescens* and a *Candida* species. When the drip site gets infected, the needle allows direct access of organisms into the vein, and the lining of the vein becomes infected. Infected emboli may then detach and go into the heart.

Of the three recent infections of which I have personal knowledge, the first was a staphylococcal septicaemia in a patient with a long plastic cannula inserted almost into the heart, which was put in to monitor central venous pressure. I have said that hyperalimentation is frequently unnecessary. The same applies to central venous pressure monitoring. It is the 'in' thing. The young housemen like to do it, though ideally the CVP line should be inserted in the operating theatre, and not in a ward. With sick patients they insert a cannula into a vein and use it not only for pressure measurements, but also for intravenous therapy, and for drug administration. CVP lines are often inserted 'just in case' and then forgotten.

Prophylactic antibiotic therapy, with ampicillin, for instance, is sometimes used in the hope of preventing infection associated with cannulae. Considering our own three organisms, namely a highly resistant *Staph. aureus*, *Serratia marcescens*, and a *Candida* species, ampicillin could encourage their growth, not prevent it, and I must strongly deprecate blind prophylactic antibiotics to cover any form of infusion therapy.

Changing the site of the needle is also important in the prevention of drip site infection. The site should be inspected every day, but this is often not done; the cannula is bound down, and no-one looks at it as long as the drip is functioning correctly. Usually the drip stops either because the site becomes infected or because the vein has leaked, and this extravasated infusion fluid is a further source of infection.

I try and encourage our junior staff to change the site of the needle, or cannula, every 48 hours. It is often very difficult, and may be impossible because, for instance, the patient has no accessible veins, or is a child. It can be difficult to re-insert the needle, but we must encourage the practice despite these difficulties.

I have been highly critical of certain of my medical colleagues, but I am as guilty as any. I have criticized the junior medical staff, but the responsibility is mine to ensure that they rotate the site of the needle and look for signs of infection. However, the nurse also has a vital part to play. A leading article in the *Lancet*, recently discussed the problem[1]. The article ended: 'The care and observation of drips is a job for nurses who understand the implications of inattention. It may be cheaper to employ the right staff than to settle an action for negligence.'

Reference

1. Leader, (1976.) *Lancet*, **i**, 291

6

The clinical manifestation of endotoxic shock arising from high level contamination
B. S. Jenkins

6.1 INTRODUCTION

'Endotoxic shock' is a disease state found in man, which bears some resemblance to the experimental endotoxic shock so extensively investigated in animals. It is important to realize that endotoxic shock as diagnosed by its clinical manifestations is not necessarily accompanied by a demonstrable bacteraemia. The endotoxin, believed to be responsible for the pathophysiology of Gram-negative bacteraemia, is a lipoprotein-carbohydrate complex found in the cell wall of the bacterium. Mice, rabbits, cats, dogs and monkeys have all been studied after the injection of endotoxin but in humans, only the intravenous infusion of heavily contaminated fluids has provided any situation analogous to the experimental work. The clinical syndromes found in man do not parallel exactly the features of experimental shock and although attempts to isolate endotoxin in human infection have been reported, at present it can only be inferred that the shock associated with Gram-negative septicaemias is due to endotoxin.

In the experimental models endotoxin appears to give rise to septic shock by the activation of two complex systems—the complement and coagulation cascades. Endotoxin provides the trigger which fires these systems to elaborate substances which have marked effects on the circulation and also provoke the syndrome of disseminated intravascular coagulation. Activation of complement also causes the release of enzymes which damage cell membranes and increase capillary permeability. An antiserum has been produced which protects animals against the lethal effects of endotoxin but only if injected before the insult.

Clinicians must constantly remind themselves that the use of the appellation 'shock' does not reveal any diagnostic insight nor does it dictate any stereotyped therapeutic manoeuvres. It merely reflects what clinical observations lead one to suppose, that inadequate tissue perfusion exists. The detailed classification of shock is beyond the scope of this paper but the following case histories exemplify those clinical features that make a clinical diagnosis of Gram-negative bacteraemia likely.

6.2 CASE HISTORIES

Case 1. A 22-year-old Chinese girl was induced with a Syntocinon drip in the 39th week of her pregnancy. The first attempt at induction was unsuccessful and the drip was discontinued. The next day the drip was restarted and within two hours she developed rigors. Three hours later her temperature rose to 40 °C. Urine and blood cultures were taken and intravenous ampicillin and clindamycin given. In the early hours of the next day she was delivered of her baby which failed to breathe. The baby was found subsequently to have pulmonary haemorrhage. Shortly after delivery the mother's blood pressure fell to 30 mm of mercury systolic. She was resuscitated with blood, large doses of steroids and was given fibrinogen. During these procedures and for 48 hours subsequently she oozed blood from all injection and venepuncture sites. Coagulation studies showed a low platelet count ($85 \times 10^9/l$), the presence of fibrin degradation products and a low fibrinogen level of $1 \cdot 3$ g/l but a normal Factor V level. Treatment with steroids and antibiotics was continued and she recovered.

A *Pseudomonas* species was recovered from the patient's blood and the Syntocinon infusion.

Comment. This case demonstrates some of the features of endotoxic shock caused by high level contamination. Initial rigors, followed by high fever and then a dramatic fall in blood pressure are highly suggestive. This patient also had some evidence of disseminated intravascular coagulation.

Case 2. Eleven days after an uneventful delivery, a 34-year-old English girl was transfused with one pint of packed red cells for anaemia. One hour after the transfusion was started she developed abdominal pain and diarrhoea and became dyspneic, cyanosed and hypotensive. A diagnosis of pulmonary embolism was made. On admission to the intensive care unit her blood pressure was 50/30 mm of mercury, the pulse rate 170 a minute and respirations were 42/minute. The central venous pressure was minus five and the pressure in the pulmonary artery was also low. Oliguria developed, she continued to pass watery stools and evidence of a coagulation disturbance (increased fibrin degradation products) was obtained. Treatment with antibiotics was started. Over the course of the next few hours she developed pulmonary edema and her heart size increased on serial chest X-rays. Her heart failure responded to treatment with digoxin and diuretics. She subsequently made a complete recovery. A *Pseudomonas* species was recovered from the patient's blood and from the packed red cells with which she was transfused.

Comment. This case is of particular interest as she developed unequivocal evidence of heart failure as one of the consequences of a massive intravenous bolus of Gram-negative organisms.

6.3 PATHOPHYSIOLOGICAL MECHANISMS

It is evident from these cases that any one individual's response to endotoxin may vary although the final outcome is diminished tissue perfusion. Four distinct patterns may be defined although any combination of these may occur concurrently.

6.3.1 Oligaemia

As a result of the endotoxic insult the integrity of the capillary membranes is destroyed and considerable quantities of proteinaceous fluid leak into the tissues. The intravascular volume falls and the effective filling pressure of the right ventricle is decreased, leading to a fall in cardiac output. The haematocrit rises and the albumin level falls. The increased capillary permeability and the lowered albumin level increase the likelihood of pulmonary edema particularly if non-protein solutions are used to restore an effective filling pressure. It is possible that massive doses of corticosteroids may have some beneficial effect on the increased capillary permeability.

6.3.2 Low venous and arterial tone

The venous reservoir which fills the right heart has a variable tone in its walls. If this tone is decreased the venous pressure will fall even in the absence of any overt change in volume. The decreased venous pressure will be accompanied by a fall in cardiac output. If, however, the resistance to left ventricular ejection is decreased simultaneously by a reduction in arteriolar tone (the systemic vascular resistance) the blood pressure will fall but the cardiac output will rise. In the early phase of Gram-negative bacteraemia, a low filling pressure, a low blood pressure but a normal or increased cardiac output are commonly seen. To some extent the fall in arteriolar resistance may represent the opening up of pre-capillary shunts. Tissue underperfusion results and the hypoxic tissues will produce lactic acid, thus causing a metabolic acidosis.

6.3.3 Intravascular coagulopathy

The precipitation of fibrin by activation of the coagulation system of the blood by endotoxin has several consequences. The red blood cells will be fragmented giving a characteristic appearance on the blood film and causing an anaemia. A marked fall in platelet count together with consumption of the components of the coagulation system will cause a severe bleeding diathesis. Widespread fibrin deposition within the capillaries will impair tissue perfusion directly.

6.3.4 Heart failure

Relatively rarely true heart failure may occur. Both right and left atrial pressures are raised and the cardiac output is decreased.

Any or all of these mechanisms if left untreated will progress to multiple organ failure and a more or less rapid progression to death.

6.4 TREATMENT

The management of endotoxic shock in our experience is most easily accomplished if these pathophysiological mechanisms are specifically defined and treated appropriately. It must be stressed that the combination of early diagnosis, removal of the source of contamination and the administration of the appropriate antibiotics are of overriding and fundamental importance.

The oligaemic syndrome, recognized by measurement of the central venous pressure, a rising haematocrit and a fall in serum albumin, requires restoration of an effective circulating volume by the use of plasma infusion. The danger of pulmonary edema must be appreciated and as previously suggested, steroids may be indicated specifically to treat the increased capillary permeability. The prognosis in this group is poor.

The patients with low venous and arterial tone have a rather better prognosis. Despite a low blood pressure organ perfusion is often maintained and therapeutic interventions to restore the blood pressure are ill advised. If a metabolic acidosis is present the use of pharmacological doses of steroids may improve true tissue flows.

In experimental animals the administration of heparin has been shown to control disseminated intravascular coagulation but in human disease it appears less effective. Its administration does require a considerable act of faith, on the present evidence, in a patient presenting with major bleeding. Fresh blood may be more appropriate.

When heart failure is found care must be taken to avoid overtransfusion and subsequent pulmonary edema particularly if there is also evidence of increased capillary permeability.

The incidence of shock lung appears remarkably low when the shock syndrome is managed according to such an analysis of the mechanisms that appear to be operative in a particular patient.

References

1. Christy, J. H. (1971). Pathophysiology of gram-negative shock. *Am. Heart J.*, **81**, 694
2. Hardaway, R. M. (1965). Microcoagulation in shock. *Am. J. Surg.*, **110**, 928
3. Lillehei, R. C., Longerbeam, J. K., Block, J. H. and Manax, W. G. (1964). Nature of irreversible shock: experimental and clinical observations. *Ann. Surg.*, **160**, 682
4. Waisbren, B. A. (1951). Bacteremia due to gram-negative bacilli other than Salmonella. *Arch. Intern. Med.*, **88**, 467
5. Weil, M. H., Shubin, H. and Biddle, M. (1964). Shock caused by gram-negative microorganisms: Analysis of 169 cases. *Ann. Intern. Med.*, **60**, 384

7

Sepsis arising from extrinsic contamination of the infusion and measures for control
D. G. Maki

7.1 BACKGROUND

Outbreaks of nosocomial septicaemia traced to intrinsic contamination of infusion products in the US and Great Britain between 1970 and 1973[1-8] have focused unprecedented attention on the iatrogenic hazards of infusion therapy, and particularly on septicaemia arising from contaminated fluid. Yet, the total number of cases identified in these outbreaks comprise but a fraction of all infusion-related septicaemias occurring in hospitals. Fortunately, commercially manufactured parenteral products which are alleged to be sterile almost inevitably are, and intrinsic contamination is exceedingly rare. The vast majority of infections associated with infusion therapy derive from extrinsic sources of contamination, with micro-organisms introduced into a previously sterile infusion or the cannula wound during therapy.

These infections are preventable. This premise forms the basis for the discussion that follows, for the goal is not to treat iatrogenic infections, but to prevent them. By critically examining existing knowledge of the reservoirs of nosocomial pathogens and their modes of transmission to the patient's infusion, it is possible to formulate rational and effective guidelines for safe administration of infusion therapy. Moreover, measures for preventing sepsis in infusion therapy arising from extrinsic sources of contamination are also effective in lessening the frequency and severity of sepsis caused by intrinsically contaminated products.

7.2 CANNULA-RELATED INFECTION

7.2.1 Plastic venous catheters

In this chapter the term 'cannula' refers to all types of plastic catheter and steel needle utilized for continuous vascular access. Plastic catheters made of polyvinylchloride, polyethylene, polypropylene, PTFE or silastic, ranging from less than 2 inches to 24 inches in length (Figure 7.1) are used in approximately one-half of all intravenous infusions in adults in the United States. Umbilical catheters in neonates will not be discussed.

7.2.1.1 *History*

It is appropriate on historical grounds to consider first of all infections arising from extrinsic contamination of intravascular cannulae and specifically, plastic catheters. Plastic catheters have been used widely since 1945. Yet as recently as 1962 the fact that they are associated with a

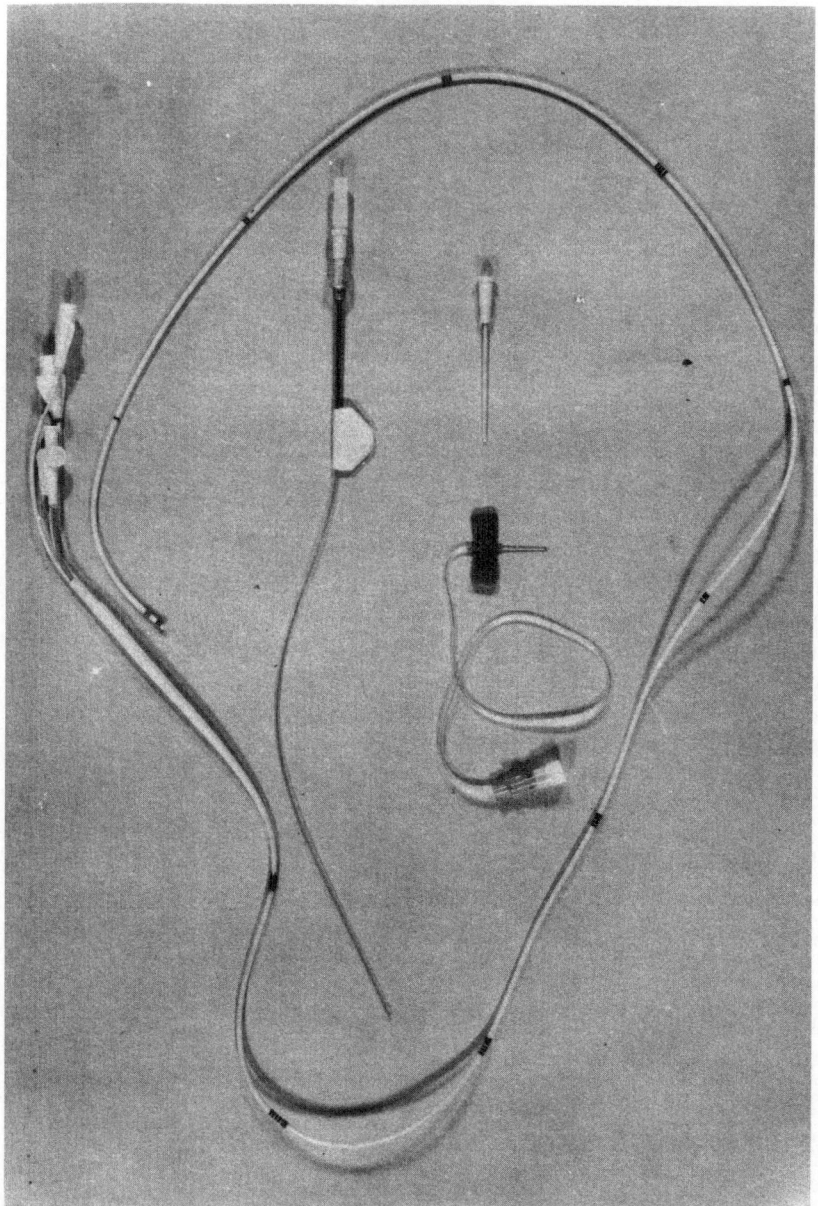

Figure 7.1 Typical vascular cannulae, including 'scalp-vein needle' (centre), 2-inch and 12-inch plastic catheters and Swan–Gonz pulmonary artery catheter (encircling all others)

significant risk of infection was largely unknown. The American Hospital Association's well-known monograph 'Control of Infections in the Hospital' in that year did not even mention intravenous therapy as a source of septicaemia and the first prospective study of catheter-related infection was not published until 1963[9]. Since that time over 40 groups of investigators have focused attention on venous catheters[8].

7.2.1.2 *Methodology of published studies and definitions*

Most studies aseptically removed venous catheters and cultured the tips qualitatively, by immersion in broth[8]. Growth was variously and generally arbitrarily designated as 'contamination', 'colonization' or 'infection'. Which designation is most appropriate is not clear in that the act of removing a catheter provides ample opportunity for contaminating it; theoretically, a single microorganism from contiguous skin flora can give a positive conventional broth culture. Moreover, microorganisms from distant sites of infection can seed the catheter tip in the absence of identified bacteraemia[9-16]. Accordingly, the pathophysiological importance and clinical interpretation of a positive catheter culture in broth has never been clear.

To implicate conclusively a catheter as a source of septicaemia has required either histological evidence of venous suppuration (which is rare) or that there is no other clinically identifiable source of infection and the blood pathogen has been isolated from no other site. These restrictions obviously limit the clinical value of a catheter culture in broth. In a later section, a new semi-quantitative method of culturing vascular catheters will be described which promises to identify catheter-related infection with considerably greater accuracy.

7.2.1.3 *Results of studies*

Rates of catheter tip cultures have ranged from 3·8 to 57% and rates of associated septicaemia from zero to as high as 8%[8]. Subclavian catheters, both for conventional infusion therapy and for total parenteral nutrition (TPN), and peripheral catheters inserted by surgical cutdown have been associated with the highest rates of septicaemia, 3·8–6·5% (Table 7.1). Steel needles, in essence 'scalp vein needles', well known for many years to paediatricians and radial artery catheters have been associated with strikingly lower rates of septicaemia, less than 1 per 500 cannulations. These observations infer the first guideline for prevention: *Infusion therapy in general and plastic catheters specifically should be employed only when clearly indicated by the patient's clinical requirements.*

TABLE 7.1 Incidence of cannula-related septicaemia with various types of cannulae

Type of cannula	Number of studies	Number of cannulations	Number of septicaemias	Incidence (%)
Conventional intraveneous therapy				
Plastic catheters*				
Percutaneous				
Peripheral	17	7618	36	0·5
Subclavian	4	393	15	3·8
Umbilical	6	374	8	2·2
Cutdowns	6	248	16	6·5
Steel needles†	5	635	1	0·2
Total parenteral nutrition (TPN)				
Centrally-placed catheters*	15	1162	139	12·0
Arterial catheters				
Radial artery	3	593	0	0
(Catheters for haemodynamic monitoring‡)				
Brachial artery§	1	619	9	1·5
(Catheters for cancer chemotherapy)				

* From published studies reviewed in Maki et al.[8]
† References 39–43 cited in text
‡ References 62–64
§ Reference 65

TABLE 7.2 Relation of duration of catheterization to results of catheter cultures and catheter-related septicaemia*

Category	Duration of catheterization (days)				
	1	2	3	≥4	Total
Number of catheters	150	288	205	273	916
Number of culture-positive (%)	28 (11·2)	70 (24·3)	56 (28·8)	91 (33·3)	245 (26·7)
Number causing septicaemias (%)	0 (—)	1 (0·3)	2 (0·7)	8 (2·9)	11 (1·2)
	1 (0·2)		10 (1·8)		

* Combined data from four published studies

Despite limitations of broth methods of culture, these many studies have been remarkably consistent on one point, that the longer catheters are left in place the higher the rates of positive cultures of catheter tips and particularly, of associated catheter-related septicaemia (Table 7.2). With cannulations exceeding 48 hours, the incidence of catheter-related septicaemia has ranged from zero to as high as 8% in individual hospitals, averaging about 2%. A cardinal guideline pertaining to the use of venous plastic catheters is obvious: *Plastic catheters, which clearly must be used in many clinical situations, should be removed whenever possible within 48 to 72 hours of insertion.* If prolonged intravenous therapy through one cannula is required in a patient with few peripheral veins, increased vigilance is demanded.

7.2.1.4 *Projections on a national scale*

If these data from a large number and wide variety of institutions are used to estimate the number of catheter-related septicaemias in the United States annually, a problem of major proportions is suggested. At least one-fourth of the 40 000 000 Americans hospitalized annually receive at least one course of infusion therapy[17], about half through plastic catheters. Conservatively estimating an overall 0·5% incidence of catheter-related septicaemia (Table 7.1) projects to 25 000 cases each year in the US.

7.2.1.5 *Pathophysiological considerations*

When a plastic catheter is inserted in a vessel a loosely organized fibrin sleeve envelops the catheter almost uniformly within 24 to 48 hours[18,19]. The catheter is a conduit directly connecting the bloodstream with the outer world and its abundant microflora. If microorganisms can reach the fibrin clot, where they are partially shielded from host defences and where high concentrations of some infusates may also hinder local defence mechanisms, they can rapidly proliferate to initiate septicaemia.

Inflammation at the catheter site (pain, swelling, redness, tenderness, lymphangitis, or a palpable cord) is extremely common in infusion therapy. Multiple physicochemical factors including catheter material and size and character of the infusate have been implicated[8,20]. Most studies have found no correlation between phlebitis and a positive catheter culture in broth, and phlebitis is present in only about half of patients with catheter-related septicaemia[8]. However, by employing a semi-quantitative method of culturing catheters, which identifies local infection, we found that catheter-related infection is strongly associated with local inflammation[21]

Moreover, during the 1970–71 US outbreak of septicaemia associated with contaminated fluids, patients with septicaemia had a much greater incidence of phlebitis than patients receiving intravenous fluids who did not develop sepsis[4]. Most patients with phlebitis obviously do not have sepsis; however, the presence of phlebitis connotes an 18-fold increased risk of concomitant or incipient catheter-induced septicaemia (Table 7.3) and augurs for immediate catheter removal.

TABLE 7.3   Relationship between infusion phlebitis and catheter-related septicaemia*

| Category | Phlebitis | |
	Absent	Present
Number of patients	995	327
Number with septicaemia	2	12†
(%)	(0·2)	(3·7)

* From five prospective studies of catheter-related infection, each reporting at least one septicaemia and complete data on phlebitis and septicaemia in all study patients[8]
† $p < 0.001$

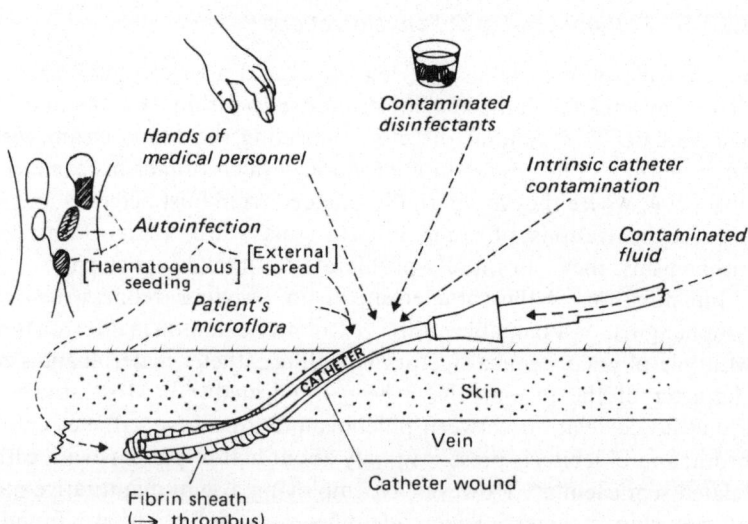

Figure 7.2   Sources of intravenous cannula-related infection

Catheter-related sepsis can derive from five possible sources of extrinsic contamination (Figure 7.2): First, the patient's own cutaneous microflora; second, the contaminated hands of medical personnel; third, contaminated disinfectants; fourth, autoinfection of the catheter wound from other un-related sites of infection; and fifth, contaminated infusion fluid. All are supported by epidemiological evidence.

7.2.1.6 *Extrinsic sources of catheter-related infection*

(a) *Cutaneous microflora of the patient and medical personnel*—The micro-biology of catheter-related infection points strongly towards skin flora of the patient and microorganisms carried on the hands of medical personnel in the genesis of these infections. *Staphylococcus epidermidis*, *Staph. aureus*, enterococcus and Gram-negative bacilli, particularly Klebsiella-Enterobacter, *Serratia*, *Pseudomonas aeruginosa* and *Acinetobacter* are recovered most frequently from positive catheter cultures; *Staph. aureus* (approximately 50%) and Gram-negative bacilli have been implicated in the majority of catheter-related septicaemias[8]. These organisms are all commonly found on the skin of hospitalized patients[22] and the hands of randomly sampled medical personnel[23,24].

A number of studies have shown a strong correlation between skin flora of the catheter site, and microorganisms recovered from catheter tips and catheter-induced septicaemia[12,14,25-27]. Cases of staphylococcal catheter-related septicaemia have been shown by phage typing to be the same strains carried by the physicians who had inserted the indicted catheters[28], and five infusion-related *Kl. pneumoniae* septicaemias in an intensive care unit were traced to contaminated hand lotions used by nurses[29] (Table 7.4).

Inadequate skin disinfection or a break in asepsis permits micro-organisms to be introduced into the wound at the time of catheter insertion or thereafter when organisms may penetrate along the interface between the catheter and tissue (Figure 7.2). Accordingly, *vigorous handwashing by the operator (or ideally the wearing of gloves) and effective cutaneous dis-infection of the insertion site (most reliably done with iodine-containing agents) are exceedingly important in the prevention of cannula-related infection.* Two percent iodine in 70% alcohol (tincture of iodine, USP) is inexpensive, well-tolerated and highly effective. Seventy percent alcohol or an iodophor are acceptable alternatives. (Critical reviews of available cutaneous antiseptics have been published[8,29a,29b]).

In general it is most prudent to view the insertion of a vascular catheter as a minor surgical procedure, in some circumstances such as in total parenteral nutrition, to the extent of using sterile drapes and gloves.

TABLE 7.4   Epidemics of infusion-related septicaemia traced to extrinsic sources of contamination

Senior author*	Years	Pathogens	Number of cases	Source
Plotkin[30]	1955–56	Ps. aeruginosa	40	Contaminated aqueous benzalkonium used to disinfect catheter sites
Malizia[31]	1960	E. cloacae	11	Same
Morse[29]	1967	Kl. pneumoniae	5	Contaminated hand lotions
Sack[32]	1968	E. cloacae and Kl. pneumoniae	5	Contaminated fluid. One (cracked?) bottle used in five consecutive patients
Phillips[33]	1970	Ps. cepacia	3	Contaminated pressure transducers for arterial pressure monitoring
Speller[34]	1970	Ps. cepacia	5	Contaminated aqueous chlorhexidine used to disinfect catheter sites
CDC[35]	1973	Flavobacterium spp.	14	Contaminated ice used to chill syringes for arterial blood gas specimen
CDC[36]	1974	Ps. cepacia	8	Contaminated aqueous benzalkonium and pressure transducers
CDC[37]	1975	Ps. cepacia and E. cloacae	5	Contaminated pressure transducers for arterial pressure monitoring
CDC[37a]	1976	E. aerogenes	7	Contaminated fluid, prepared in central pharmacy. Use of same syringe to add KCl to multiple units of D5%/0·2 NS

* Cited sources conform to text references

Catheters inserted under less than optimal conditions of asepsis, for instance during emergency resuscitations, and malfunctioning catheters (leaking, occluded, infiltrated or especially those associated with phlebitis) are more likely to be culture-positive and cause septicaemia and should be promptly replaced. Venous pressure monitoring also increases the incidence of positive catheter cultures[16] and should never be done with catheters used for total parenteral nutrition which are uniquely susceptible to producing sepsis (Table 7.1).

(b) *Autoinfection*—Catheters inserted in patients with active infections such as those of the urinary tract, a surgical wound or pneumonia, become culture positive more frequently than catheters in non-infected patients[12-14]. Organisms from the infection are transmitted to the infusion site or contaminate the operator's hands and enter the catheter wound at the time of insertion or during subsequent manipulations by personnel or even the patient. However, bacteraemic seeding almost certainly occurs as well. Henzel[13] reported eight cases of catheter-related septicaemia which followed by 8-15 days bacteraemic infections with the same organism arising from sites of infection unrelated to the infusion. Presumably these catheters which were in place at the time of the initial bacteraemia became haematogenously colonized and subsequently gave rise to catheter-related septicaemia. *Meticulous asepsis in catheter care is of even greater importance in infected patients.* Vascular catheters present during culture-proven septicaemia, particularly if already in place for prolonged periods and likely to have a substantial enveloping fibrin sheath, should be replaced to prevent colonization and later secondary sepsis.

(c) *Contaminated disinfectants*—Ten epidemics of infusion-related septicaemia originating from extrinsic sources of contamination have been reported[29,30-37a] (Table 7.4). Three outbreaks have implicated chemical skin disinfectants heavily contaminated (when quantified, $> 10^5$/ml) by Gram-negative bacilli. These were due to aqueous benzalkonium[30,31] (which is readily inactivated by contact with cellulose fibres or protein[38]) and aqueous chlorhexidine[34] (which also supports growth of *Pseudomonas* under conditions of alkalinity[38a]). Preparing the catheter site with a contaminated solution is not unlike rinsing it with grossly infected urine. *Aqueous solutions of benzalkonium or chlorhexidine* should not be used for disinfection in infusion therapy* (or anywhere else for that matter where the failure of disinfection will be catastrophic).

(d) *Contaminated infusion fluid*—Septicaemia caused by contaminated fluid is not truly cannula-related and usually produces a more fulminant clinical picture of endotoxaemia than catheter-related infection[1-8,32]. However, levels of fluid contamination too low to give clinical symptoms in theory can colonize the fibrin sheath enveloping the catheter, hereby producing true catheter-related septicaemia. Measures for prevention of extrinsic contamination of infusion fluid are considered in a subsequent section.

---

* A 70% *alcoholic* solution (tincture) of chlorhexidine digluconate ('Hibitane') appears to be highly effective and relatively safe[29a]

7.2.2 Steel needles

Although controlled comparative studies have not been performed, steel needles (in the USA synonymous with 'scalp-vein needles') appear to be much safer than plastic catheters in regard to infection (Table 7.1). Only one case of needle-related septicaemia was identified in 635 patients in five prospective studies[39-43]. Moreover, steel needles caused substantially less phlebitis than plastic catheters, even with comparable periods of placement. Possible reasons for the apparent greater safety of steel needles have been considered in a prior review[8].

The shorter (up to 7 cm) and smaller-bore plastic catheters made of Teflon rather than polyethylene or polyvinylchloride, now used widely in the USA, may be substantially safer in regard to infection than the large polyethylene and polyvinylchloride catheters employed in most published studies of catheter-related sepsis. These smaller catheters might even be as safe as steel needles. However, until comparative studies are done, steel needles must be regarded as the safest type of cannula for general use.

Without question plastic catheters are mandatory in certain well-defined clinical circumstances such as central venous pressure monitoring, total parenteral nutrition and when a secure route of access is required for critically ill patients. But *for elective infusions steel needles should be used whenever feasible in preference to plastic catheters.*

It should be pointed out that there have been five reported cases of septicaemia caused by steel needles[39,44,45]; three occurred in patients with cancer including one case of suppurative phlebitis[45]. Thus, all types of cannulae carry some risk and should be regarded as potential avenues for infection.

7.2.3 Suppurative phlebitis

This entity (also commonly referred to as septic thrombophlebitis) is the most dread and extreme form of cannula-related infection. The vein becomes an endovascular abscess, engorged by grossly infected pus, discharging massive numbers of microorganisms into the blood stream (Figure 7.3). Understandably, the most common manifestation is a refractory and often overwhelming septicaemia. Coagulase-positive *Staph. aureus,* and since the late 1960s, multiply-resistant Gram-negative bacilli, especially Klebsiella-Enterobacter, *Pseudomonas* and *Serratia,* and *Candida* have been most frequently implicated[45-54].

With rare exception[45] suppurative phlebitis has usually derived from plastic catheters left in place for more than 48 hours. Most reports have

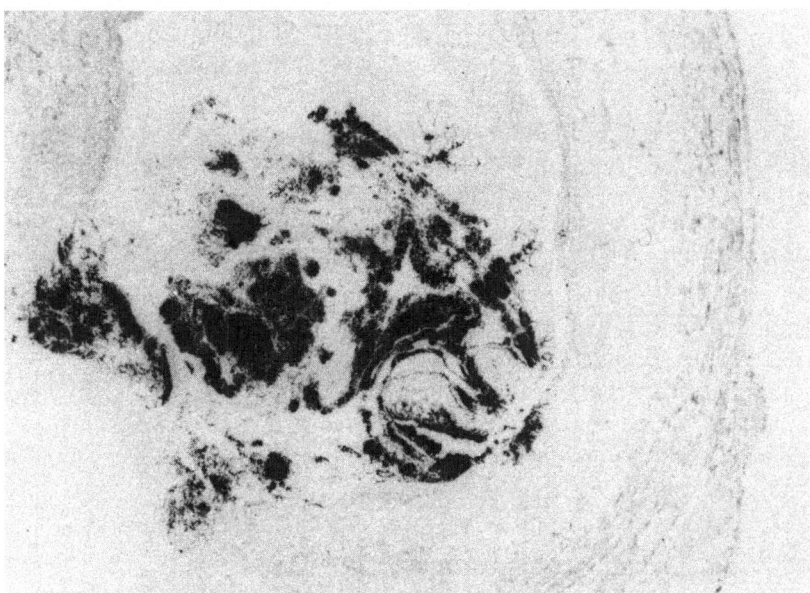

Figure 7.3 Histopathology of vein involved by suppurative phlebitis (Gomori-Methenamine Silver × 40). Black masses are *Candida* colonies infiltrating intra-luminal thrombus and the vessel wall

been from burn centres. Patients with full thickness burns are uniquely susceptible, probably because of first, the massive population of surface microorganisms which can colonize the catheter wound directly or the catheter thrombus by bacteraemic spread, second, an intrinsic hyper-coagulable state, third, masking of local signs and symptoms of catheter-related infection by concurrent burn wound infection and fourth, limited sites for vascular access, both of the latter implicity delaying cannula removal. Suppurative phlebitis rivals infection of the burn wound as a cause of fatal infection in the burn patient at the present time[47,54].

Warden and his co-workers[51] recently reported 25 instances in 139 burn patients of septic thrombosis of the central great veins, specifically involving the superior vena cava (three cases), the subclavian vein (nine cases) or ileofemoral vein (13 cases), all associated with indwelling plastic catheters used for total parenteral nutrition, venous pressure monitoring or conventional infusion therapy. Only three cases were detected ante-mortem. Secondary septic pulmonary emboli were present in half the cases. Even more recently, Popp and his co-workers in the Cincinatti

Shriners Burn Institute reported 16 cases of bacteraemia and fungaemia related to catheters used for total parenteral nutrition in burned children, including five cases of fatal superior vena caval septic thrombosis[54]. All of these latter cases occurred in patients with full-thickness burns involving the subclavian area, necessitating central venous cannulation through peripheral veins or the burn wound. Moreover, all five cases had bacterial endocarditis, four with *Candida*, at autopsy.

In a recent prospective study in the University of Wisconsin Burn Unit[55], every vascular cannula was cultured semi-quantitatively[21]. Six patients with burns ranging from 30 to 90% of the body surface (mean, 57%) which limited vascular access to veins of the lower extremities suffered five episodes of catheter-related septicaemia, three associated with suppurative phlebitis.

In patients without burns, suppurative phlebitis appears to be much more frequent in cannulations of veins of the lower extremities[8]. *Venous cannulation of the lower extremity in adults should be avoided.*

7.2.4 Topical antimicrobial drugs

Catheter-related sepsis would be greatly minimized if catheters could be removed without fail within 48 hours but this is not always feasible in patients with limited peripheral veins who must have a secure route for venous access. The great majority of catheter-related septicaemias arise from extrinsic microorganisms that infect the wound first, as shown by the strong association which exists between microorganisms present on skin surrounding the catheter site and organisms causing catheter-related septicaemia[12,14,25-27], by hospitals which utilize iodine-containing agents for cutaneous disinfection with a formal programme for catheter care who report substantially lower rates of catheter-related sepsis[8], and by the catheter-related septicaemias which have been traced to physician-carriers of coagulase-positive staphylococci[28], or to contaminated hand lotions used by nurses[29] and to contaminated skin antiseptics[30,31,34] (Table 7.4). Thus in theory application of a topical antimicrobial agent to the catheter wound should confer some degree of protection against extrinsic con-tamination and infection. However, the six studies published to date[10,56-60] have yielded conflicting results, probably because of the limited number of catheters (and bacteraemias) in each. Combining the results of four studies which all used the same antibiotic combination (polymyxin, neomycin and bacitracin)[10,56-58] suggests a beneficial effect (Table 7.5). However, topical antibiotics may promote superinfection by resistant Gram-negative bacilli or yeasts; *Candida* was recovered from catheters in place more than

72 hours only in patients receiving topical antibiotics. Topical antiseptics such as iodophors which are already widely used in many US programmes for total parenteral nutrition could possibly obviate this hazard. More comprehensive studies are urgently needed in this area. *Application of a topical combination antibiotic or antiseptic ointment to the cannula site at the time of insertion and at periodic intervals thereafter may confer added protection against infection.*

TABLE 7.5 **Influence of topical antimicrobial agents in prevention of catheter-related septicaemia***

	Treatment group	
Category	*Control*	*Antimicrobial agents*
Number of patients	581	514
Number of septicaemias	9	2†
(%)	(1·5)	(0·4)

* From four prospective studies[10,56−58] which all used a commercial preparation containing polymyxin, neomycin and bacitracin

† $p < 0.05$

7.2.5 Infection due to arterial catheters

In the past decade there has been a marked upsurge in the use of indwelling arterial catheters for haemodynamic and blood-gas monitoring. Moreover, direct perfusion of tumours by selective intra-arterial infusion of anti-neoplastic drugs is now an established method for treatment of non-resectable malignant masses.

7.2.5.1 *Radial artery catheters*

Although a single reported case of septic endarteritis was reported in 1970[61], no study specifically examined the risk of systemic infection with indwelling radial arterial catheters until 1974. Gardner, *et al.*[62] found eight positive radial artery catheters of 200 cultured in an 11 month prospective study, though none were associated with local infection or septicaemia. However, most catheters were in place for 4 days or less. Two other reports of experience with these catheters did not specifically examine infection, but clinically did not identify any septicaemias which could be attributed to the catheter[63,64].

The apparently greater immunity of radial artery catheters to infection compared with indwelling venous catheters (Table 7.1) may be related in part first, to the more rapid rate of arterial blood flow, second, to the routine use of heparin with arterial catheters, lessening local thrombogenesis, third, to the anatomically deeper (and more protected) location of arteries compared with veins, and fourth, to the routine use of gloves and the generally greater attention paid to local asepsis during arterial catheter insertion.

Recently three outbreaks of septicaemia have been traced to extrinsic contamination of transducers used for arterial pressure monitoring[33,36,37] and one outbreak to contaminated ice used to chill syringes used for obtaining arterial blood-gas specimens[35] (Table 7.4). These outbreaks were caused by Gram-negative bacilli with growth potential in fluid and their implications in terms of prevention will be discussed in a subsequent section.

7.2.5.2 *Arterial catheters for cancer chemotherapy*

Between January and April 1974, three patients in our institution developed staphylococcal endarteritis in association with percutaneous brachial artery catheters used for cancer chemotherapy. No common phage-type was found. Retrospective review of our experience with this mode of therapy over the past four years identified nine septicaemias ($1 \cdot 5 \%$ of all catheterizations) clearly related to the catheter[65]. All were caused by *Staph. aureus*. Difficult cannulations or the need for catheter repositioning, radiotherapy and increased patient debilitation (as manifested by hypoalbuminaemia or leukopaenia) were all strongly associated with an increased risk of septicaemia when compared with an uninfected control group also receiving intra-arterial chemotherapy. Duration of cannulation did not influence susceptibility to infection; infected patients became symptomatic within 4–20 (mean $9 \cdot 0$) days as compared to a mean $18 \cdot 0$ days of cannulation in a non-infected control group, pointing to the importance of host factors and excessive manipulation of the catheter in susceptibility to these infections. A formal programme for catheter care was instituted, including a pre-insertion hexachlorophene shower and scrub of the cannulation site, together with periodic application of a combination antibiotic ointment. Now, no infections have occurred in the past 12 months in over 150 patients who have received intra-arterial chemotherapy.

7.2.6 Semi-quantitative method of culturing vascular catheters

As previously noted, considerable evidence suggests that most catheter-related septicaemias begin as local infections of the catheter wound. Quantitative culture of materials from the catheter tract or culture of the outer surface of the catheter should reflect the microbiological status of the wound.

We have developed and clinically tested a semi-quantitative (SQ) method for culturing vascular catheters and recently reported our experience in 198 patients[21]. The amputated catheter segment distal to the skin surface is rolled back and forth across the surface of a blood agar plate, then immersed in broth. Ninety percent of 250 catheters were SQ culture-negative, yielding no growth whatsoever, growth only in broth or only 1–7 colonies on the plate; none were associated with septicaemia. In contrast, 10% of catheters gave heavy growth on the plate (SQ-positive); septicaemia originated from four of these 25 catheters ($p = 0.008$). Moreover, in contrast to results with the broth method in most studies[8], positivity by SQ culture was strongly associated with local inflammation ($p < 0.001$). None of 37 catheters exposed *in situ* to bacteraemia from sites of infection unrelated to the catheter were SQ-positive with the blood stream pathogen whereas four yielded matching growth in broth.

This SQ method differentiates catheter-related infection from contamination with greater accuracy than conventional broth culture. Moreover, microbiological identification of isolates and susceptibility testing are accelerated. The method also shows considerable promise for earlier identification of suppurative phlebitis[55] and for studies of new techniques of local asepsis in catheter care.

7.3. EXTRINSIC CONTAMINATION OF INFUSION FLUID

7.3.1 Historical background

Michaels and Ruebner[66] in 1953 reported two cases of coliform septicaemia which they attributed to contaminated infusion fluid because in both cases the infecting organism was recovered in heavy numbers from the in-use administration set. Despite the startling implications of this paper, the potential for contamination for infusion fluid was unmentioned in the medical literature until Wilmore and Dudrick in 1969 reported their experience with an in-line membrane filter[67]. In 1970, two reports of bacteraemic infections aetiologically implicated extrinsic contamination of infusion fluid[32,68]. In one incident, five consecutive patients developed severe Gram-negative septicaemia postoperatively; all had received succinylcholine in 5 % dextrose in Ringer's solutions from a single bottle[32] (Table 7.4). Entry through a crack was hypothesized based on findings in a subsequent sixth case. In 1971 Duma and his co-workers reported four cases of infusion-related septicaemia with in-use infusion fluid con-

TABLE 7.6   Studies of in-use contamination of conventional intravenous fluid

Senior author*	Year	Fluid brand	Type container	Number Units sampled	Prevalence (%) contamination Gram-neg.	Overall
Deeb[73]	1971	NS†	Bottle	321	2·2	3·8
Duma[69]	1971	Abbott	Bottle	68	6	13‡
Maki[70]	1971	Baxter	Bottle	94	2	11
Maki[71]	1971	Abbott	Bottle	135	8·8	20·0 ⎫ §
		Cutter	Bottle	148	2·0	6·8 ⎭
Phillips[5]	1972	Hospital-made	Bottle	33	30	30ᶜ
Colvin[15]	1972	Baxter	Bottle	38	0	0
Letcher[74]	1972	Travenol	Bag	366	0	10·4
Collin[75]	1973	NS	Bottle	50	1	3
Enerot[76]	1973	NS	Bottle	171	0	2·9
Steckel[77]	1973	NS	Bottle	549	0	1·6
Ravin[78]	1974	Travenol	Bag	906	1·7	4·0
Woodside[78a]	1975	NS	Bottle	952	NS	4·7
			Bag	51	NS	0

* Cited sources conform to text references
† Not stated
‡ Multiple sites of infusion apparatus cultured; only results of fluid culture tabulated here
§ Comparative study in one hospital during US epidemic caused by intrinsically contaminated Abbott products[1-4]; patients received one or the other brand by random allocation
ᶜ Ongoing epidemic caused by intrinsic contamination with *Ps. thomasii*

taminated by organisms identical to those isolated from blood[69]. Thirty-five percent of 68 in-use systems in their hospital contained contaminants, including the fluid within 13 % of administration sets (Table 7.6). The high prevalence of contamination and the resulting four infections were attributed to manipulations of the infusion apparatus in the course of therapy. In 1970–71, the potential for disease from contaminated infusate became dramatically apparent when many hospitals throughout the United States experienced outbreaks of nosocomial septicaemia traced to the intrinsically contaminated products of one manufacturer, Abbott Laboratories[1-4]. Since 1971 three additional outbreaks of septicaemia associated with contaminated fluids have been caused by intrinsically contaminated products[5-7]; extrinsic contamination of the fluid delivery system resulted in epidemics in four hopsitals[33,36-37a] (Table 7.4).

7.3.2   Studies of extrinsic contamination of fluid

A major fall-out of the large 1970–71 US outbreak was the realization that even if fluid is sterile when it arrives from the manufacturer, it can readily become contaminated from extrinsic sources during use in the hospital. Our studies of the in-use products of two other manufacturers (Cutter and Baxter Laboratories) in early 1971 found that 6·8–11% of infusion systems in use in the hospital at any time contained microorganisms[70,71] (Table 7.6). In both studies, contamination was very low level (Table 7.7) and primarily with microorganisms regarded as skin commensals which grow poorly, if at all, in glucose-containing fluids (*Staph. epidermidis*, *Bacillus* spp. and diphtheroids). Only members of

TABLE 7.7   **Levels of in-use contamination of infusion fluid—two hospital surveys**

| Count* (Number of organisms/infusion) | Number of contaminated infusions, by brand | | |
| | Comparative study (Feb. 1971)† | | |
	Abbott	Cutter	Baxter‡
0	108	138	84
1	7	7	5
3–10	11	1	3
11–20	2	1	1
20–99	2		
> 100	5	1	1
Total with > 1 organism	27	10	10
(Prevalence, %)	(20·0)	(6·8)	(11)

* By membrane filtration of remaining contents of bottles and/or administration sets
† During 1970–71 outbreak of septicaemia traced to instrinsic contamination of Abbott's infusion systems[1-4]. Relative contributions of intrinsic contaminants and contamination introduced during clinical use (extrinsic) is not known. From Maki, D. G., Sher, N. and Mandel, G. Unpublished data
‡ From Maki *et al.*[70]

tribe Klebsielleae (*Klebsiella, Enterobacter,* and *Serratia*) were recovered in large numbers. (This observation and the predominance of *Enterobacter* spp. in the ongoing epidemic were explained by our *in vitro* studies of microbial growth in infusion fluid[72] (discussed in Chapter 2)). In both studies contamination appeared to be of extrinsic origin, related to the many manipulations of systems which comprise infusion therapy. An important observation of Duma's[69] and these studies[70,71] was that the presence of contamination was directly related to the duration of uninterrupted infusion, suggesting that the risk of contamination is cumulative (Table 7.8). Systems in continuous use beyond 48 hours were more frequently contaminated than systems in use less than 48 hours, a relationship very similar to that governing extrinsic contamination of venous catheters.

TABLE 7.8   Relationship of duration of infusion therapy and in-use contamination of infusion fluid*

Duration of continuous infusion therapy	No. systems at risk	No. (%) with fluid contamination
≤48 hours	33	1 (3)
>48 hours	61	9 (15)

* From Maki *et al.*[70]

TABLE 7.9   Studies of in-use contamination of total parenteral nutrition fluid

Senior author*	Year	Fluid brand	Number infusions sampled	Prevalence (%) contamination	
				Candida	Overall
Wilmore[67]	1969	NS†	250	NS	2·8
Deeb[73]	1971	NS	85	25	38
Asch[79]	1972	Baxter, Cutter	82	0	39
Sanderson[80]	1973	NS	706	0	2·1
Steckel[77]	1973	Baxter	69	0	6
Miller[81]	1973	Baxter	1902‡	0·5	7·9
Miller[82]	1975	Baxter	4848‡	0·7	7·5
Popp[54]	1974	Abbott, Cutter	51	0	2

* Cited sources conform to text references
† Not stated
‡ From 3 to 9 separate specimens (fluid and membrane filters) from each infusion were cultured; each specimen is tabulated separately in this table. In two studies, 361–680 infusions in 20–22 patients were cultured serially

These early studies have been confirmed in a number of other centres[5,15,73-78a] (Table 7.6). About 5% of in-use infusions contain microorganisms, usually in very low numbers. About 1-2%, on the average contain viable Gram-negative bacilli that might have growth potential in the fluid. Except for one study[73], investigators examining TPN solutions in-use found little contamination in general, or *Candida* specifically[54,67,73,77,79-82] (Table 7.9).

7.3.3 Significance of extrinsic contamination

Contamination of infusion fluid from extrinsic sources has probably caused sporadic septicaemias for as long as infusion therapy has been employed. However, with rare exceptions[32,66,68,69] the association with contaminated fluid has for the most part remained unrecognized or the infection has been attributed to the cannula.

The incidence of *infection* caused by extrinsic contamination of fluid is unknown at the present time. It is probably substantially lower than the incidence of catheter-related septicaemia. Most studies of catheter-related infection found 1-5% of randomly sampled catheters were associated with septicaemia[8] (Table 7.1). Twenty studies of comparable size listed in Tables 7.6 and 7.9, which cultured infusate during use detected only five septicaemias related to contamination among over 6000 infusions sampled, an incidence of 0·1%. However, this comparison is compromised by the fact that the majority of these studies of in-use fluid were carried out in hospitals following the recommendation that all delivery apparatus be empirically replaced every 24–48 hours. As will be discussed, this measure diminishes the likelihood of contaminants propagating to levels which can cause septicaemia. Thus, as long as this guideline is followed widely, the 'potential' incidence of septicaemia arising from extrinsically contaminated fluid will remain conjectural.

The most fruitful approach to determine the current incidence of septicaemia caused by extrinsically contaminated fluids would be always to culture infusion fluid whenever a patient receiving intravenous therapy develops clinical signs of sepsis.

7.3.4 Mechanisms of extrinsic contamination

7.3.4.1 *General considerations*

In theory, any manipulation of the infusion system (Figure 7.4) in compounding the admixture, attaching the administration set, administration

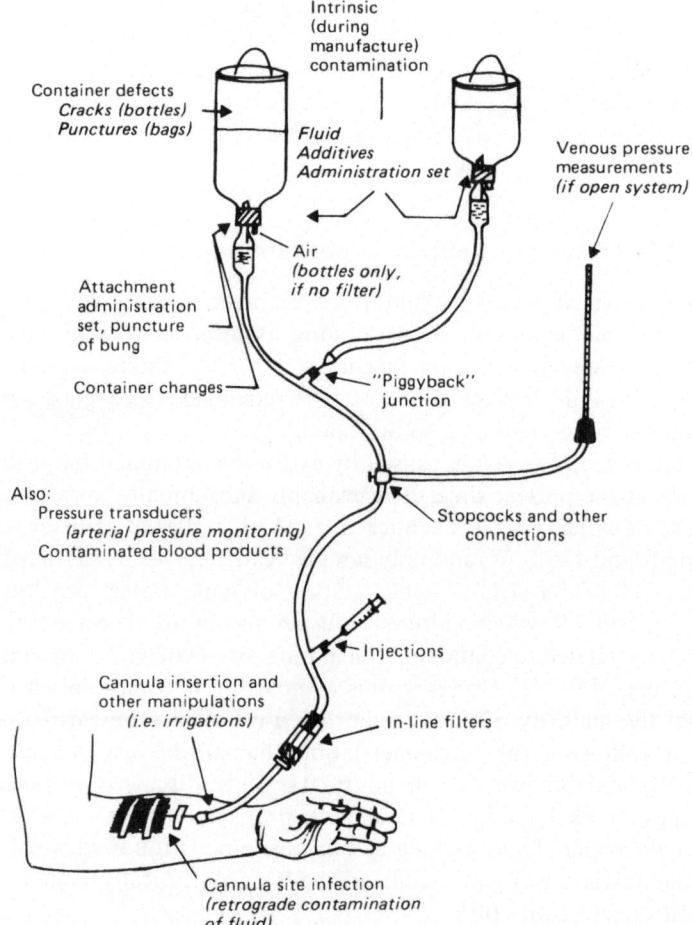

Figure 7.4   Potential sources for contamination of infusion fluid

of blood products, adding medications to the container, manipulations of stopcocks and other junctions, injection into the line, or manipulations of the cannula, can insinuate microorganisms into fluid. However, the relative importance of each of these is unknown. In-use contamination is sufficiently infrequent that quantifying the specific risk of each individual manipulations, especially with statistical significance, would require study of an astronomical number of systems. Yet, some general conclusions can be inferred from available data.

7.3.4.2 *Specific factors*

(a)   *Type of container*—Clinical[69,71]   (Table   7.7)   and   laboratory[2,83,84,84a,84b] studies and the large 1970–71 US outbreak[1–4] have
demonstrated conclusively that the open system utilizing a threaded
screw-cap closure (no longer used for infusion products in the US) is
substantially more hazardous than the closed system with a rubber bung
closure and piercing pin connector. However, three outbreaks due to
intrinsic contamination in a bung closure system[5–7] have amply demonstrated that no specific design should automatically be assumed safe.

The natural rubber used for bung closures has been shown to be a
source of contamination in the past. Fungi were found in about half of
sampled bottles in a 1966 Australian study although clinical correlations
were not provided[85]; 'coring of contaminated blisters' on the bung was
postulated to be the mechanisms of entry. All US manufacturers now
utilize coated bungs and this form of contamination is presumably no
longer a problem.

There is insufficient evidence to state whether the various commercial
brands specifically, or bottle and flexible plastic (bag) containers in general,
all of which employ a piercing pin connector, vary significantly in their
susceptibility to contamination (Tables 7.6, 7.9 and 7.10). Three studies
suggest that plastic bags may be at greater risk of becoming contaminated
in-use than closed, bottle systems[74,86,87]. However, Woodside *et al.*
found no in-use contamination of fluid in 51 plastic containers in contrast
to a 4·7% rate of contamination in 952 glass bottles[78a] and a simulation
study by McAllister and his co-workers showed a markedly lower rate of
in-use contamination of 'minibags' (0·7%) used for intermittent administration of intravenous medications, as compared with 'minibottles'
(7·1%) and in-line burettes (12·9%)[88]. Clearly, larger, well-controlled
comparative studies will be required to conclusively determine the influence
of design on vulnerability to contamination.

(b)   *Contaminated air*—Perceval[89], Arnold and Hepler[90], and Hansen
and Hepler[91] in simulation studies have demonstrated that fluid can
become contaminated by the influx of unfiltered air when bottles (which
normally have a vacuum over the fluid) are prepared and administered. Most
manufacturers now incorporate a filter over the air vent of bottles to obviate
this potential hazard. Fluid within plastic bags is not subject to this risk.

Hospital air contains relatively few Gram-negative bacilli or *Candida*[92].
Thus, it is unlikely that airborne contaminants, even in the absence of
vent filters, pose much of a clinical hazard, although obviously every
effort should be made to prevent contamination from any source.

TABLE 7.10 Studies of contamination of infusion fluid immediately after compounding, before clinical use

Type of infusion fluid	Senior author*	Year	Brand	Type container	No. units sampled	Prevalence (%) contamination		
						Gram-neg. bacilli	Candida	Overall
Conventional	Miller[86]	1971	Abbott	Bottle	NS†	NS	NS	16·2
			Baxter	Bottle	NS	NS	NS	8·4
			Travenol	Bag	NS	NS	NS	17·7
	Buth[93]	1973	Travenol	Bag	492	0	0	1·4
	Steckel[77]	1973	NS	NS	549	0	0	1·6
	Kundsin[94]	1973	Travenol	Bag	679	0	0	0·9
	Poretz[87]	1974	Travenol	Bag	54	2·0	0	5·6
			Baxter	Bottle	55	0	0	5·5
	Hanson[95]	1974	Abbott	Bottle	155	0	0	5·2
	McAllister[88]	1974	Travenol	Bottle (burette)	144	0	0	12·9
				Mini bottle	144	0	0	7·1
				Mini bag	144	0	0	0·7
Total parenteral nutrition	Hak[96]	1971	Abbott	Bottle	1078	0·4	0·1	2·5
	Ryan[97]	1972	NS	Bottle	approx. 1000	0	0	0
	Copeland[98]	1974	NS	Bottle	1017	NS	NS	3·0

* Cited sources conform to text references
† Not stated

(c) *Defects in the container*—As previously described, a cracked bottle was postulated to be the mode of microbial contamination in a cluster of five Gram-negative bacillary septicaemias reported by Sack[32]. In that same year, Robertson reported two instances of visible contamination of fluid by *Trichoderma* spp. and *Penicillium* spp. which were associated with minute cracks in the bottles[68]. One patient experienced transient fungaemia. *Thus, fluid containers, bottles or bags, should be examined carefully before use and discarded if defects such as cracks or leaks or if cloudiness or precipitates are detected. Bottles lacking a vacuum should also be discarded.* (However, as emphasized in Chapter 2, absence of macroscopic abnormality does not guarantee freedom from fluid contamination.)

(d) *Compounding the admixture*—The rates of contamination of fluid sampled immediately after compounding[77,86-88,93-98] (Table 7.10), even in the pharmacy under laminar flow hoods, do not differ significantly from rates of contamination of in-use fluid on the ward (Table 7.6). Thus, preparation of the admixture constitutes a significant source of extrinsic contamination. Moreover, if contamination occurs here, microorganisms are inoculated into the container which is a stagnant reservoir where organisms with growth potential in fluid probably pose the greatest hazard. *Fluid admixtures should be used immediately after compounding and no bottle or bag should hang for over 24 hours.*

(e) *Additives*—Although additives themselves can be contaminated[99] and the act of introducing additives into the bottle or administration set can introduce contamination, the published studies are inconclusive. Kundsin *et al.*[94] cultured fluid immediately after attachment of the administration set (before clinical use) and found the rate of contamination to be directly proportional to the number of additives in the admixture. D'Arcy and Woodside were able to culture microorganisms from 56% of containers with additives, but only 12% without added medications[100], but this group found a much more marginal difference (6·7% v. 3·9%) in a later, much larger study[78a]. Five other culture surveys have found little correlation between presence of additives and contamination of fluid[70,74,76,86,95]. Much larger studies would be required to determine conclusively the clinical hazard of additives.

(f) *Stopcocks and connectors*—In theory in-line junctions would appear to be prominent portals for contamination to enter the system, particularly since they are handled so frequently. Moreover, stopcocks are often grossly soiled by dried fluid or blood. Yet, Duma *et al.* cultured the injection ports of administration sets and found very infrequent contamination by Gram-negative bacilli, concluding that these ports were an infrequent source of hazardous contamination[69]. McArthur and her co-workers cultured the inner surfaces of stopcock connectors and found 2% contaminated with Gram-negative bacilli[101]. Fluid was not cultured and no clinical correlations were reported. A number of total parenteral nutrition programmes routinely wipe all connectors with disinfectants before reattaching, however the value of this measure is unknown, the added manipulation might paradoxically even increase the risk of extrinsic contamination. In general, stopcocks and junctions such as 'piggyback' Y-connections using a needle should be kept to a minimum.

(g) *Blood products*—From 1 to 6% of blood units have been found to contain bacteria[102–103], yet clinical infection has been rare. This is probably because blood products are refrigerated so that contamination is of very low level and because most medical personnel are aware that blood products must be infused promptly upon arrival from the blood bank. Occasional septicaemias traced to contaminated blood have been characterized by severe septic shock with a high mortality[104,105]. Psychrophilic (cold growing) organisms, usually pseudomonads, *Serratia* or coliforms (Table 7.13), have been implicated and bacteria were usually visible on direct Gram-stained smear of the involved blood product. Recently outbreaks of sepsis due to *E. cloacae*[103] and *Salm. choleraesuis*[106] were traced to contaminated platelet pools which are commonly stored at 25 °C to prolong viability. *Blood products should be infused as promptly as possible once prepared.* Also, because small quantities of blood greatly broaden the spectrum of microorganisms capable of growth in fluid[72], upon completion of a blood transfusion the entire delivery apparatus should be changed.

(h) *Retrograde contamination*—Fluid can become contaminated by microorganisms on the cannula tip by retrograde spread up the tubing[81,82,107,108]. It has been shown *in vitro* that microorganisms can ascend more than 1·5 metres against a continuous flow of fluid[109]. Backup of blood into the tubing, associated with filter malfunction[107] or accidental disconnection[108] has resulted in contamination of fluid by *Candida*, also recovered from the catheter and from blood cultures. Yet, in five studies of in-line membrane filters, microorganisms were found on the patient side of the filter far less frequently than above it[67,79,81,82,110]. The largest of these studies by Miller and Grogan[82], which incorporated three filters into each patients system, concluded that reflux as a source of contamination was rare.

(i) *Arterial pressure transducers*—Three outbreaks have stemmed from extrinsic contamination of transducers used for arterial pressure monitoring[33,36,37] (Table 7.4). Three features of these monitoring systems increase the hazard of contaminated fluid, firstly, the infusion usually runs very slowly, secondly, blood commonly refluxes back into the line, and thirdly, the system is heavily manipulated by medical personnel (obtaining, for instance, blood specimens or irrigating the catheter). The fact that saline is a poor growth medium for most microorganisms (Chapter 2) probably prevents most extrinsic contaminants from reaching dangerous levels unless the inoculum is very large, as probably occurred in these outbreaks. *The entire infusion apparatus (fluid containers and lines) of cardiovascular monitoring systems should be replaced every 24–48 hours. Pressure transducers should be sterilized with ethylene oxide or glutaraldehyde and changed as frequently as possible.* Quaternary ammonium disinfectants or aqueous chlorhexidine which caused one and perpetuated two outbreaks by their ineffectiveness against Gram-negative bacilli, should not be employed.

(j) *Administration sets*—The administration set (drip set; giving set) is probably manipulated more frequently than any other part of the infusion system. Duma *et al.* first focused attention on the vulnerability of administration sets to extrinsic contamination, particularly volume reservoirs (burettes) used for administration of intravenous drugs[69]. In the 1970–71 US outbreak we found that the mean length of time the bottle had been hanging at the onset of septicaemia and the mean number of hours the patients had received continuous infusion therapy through the same administration set were both considerably longer in septicaemia cases as compared with uninfected recipients of intravenous therapy on the same hospital units[4]. Until 1971 administrations sets were not routinely changed every 24–48 hours and they were usually replaced only when they malfunctioned or became grossly soiled and aesthetically offensive. Michaels and Ruebner first demonstrated[66], and it has been subsequently confirmed[8], that microorganisms capable of growth in the fluid, once introduced into an in-use system, can perpetuate in the administration set for days despite serial replacements of the fluid container.

(k) *The 24–48-hour set change recommendation*—In view of the cumulative nature of in-use contamination of fluid (Table 7.8), whether of intrinsic[4] or extrinsic origin[69–71,74], and the ability of many common hopsital pathogens to amplify this contamination exponentially, *it is recommended that the entire delivery system down to the cannula (containers and administration sets) be routinely changed every 24–48 hours and at each change of cannula all equipment be totally replaced*; bottles should be changed with the administration set. Several hospitals instituting this control measure in the 1970–71 US outbreak caused by intrinsically contaminated products experienced a significant decrease in epidemic septicaemias[1–4]. The efficacy of this simple measure in lessening infections due to intrinsic contamination reinforces its value for prevention of infections caused by extrinsically introduced organisms.

The cost of this empirical control measure on a national scale is obviously substantial. In that extrinsic contamination, particularly by organisms able to grow in fluid is relatively infrequent and the incidence of sepsis caused by extrinsic contamination is probably quite low (1 per 1000 infusion days or less), the cost-benefit of routine set changing remains to be determined, and in particular, if it is to be done, the choice of the most economical yet effective interval. Studies on a very large scale, encompassing thousands of infusions will be required to ascertain whether 24 hours, 48 hours or even longer is the optimal period for routinely replacing the delivery apparatus. Until such studies are performed, 24–48 hours seems most prudent.

7.3.4.2 *Summary pertaining to modes of contamination*

The majority of microorganisms recovered from in-use fluids are common skin flora including Gram-negative bacilli which as previously noted are present in high frequency on the skin of patients[22] and the hands of up to 80% of hospital personnel[23,24]. Fluid is probably most likely to become contaminated when the concentration of extrinsic microorganisms is heaviest, for instance, *Kl. pneumoniae* infusion-associated septicaemias in an intensive care unit linked to heavily contaminated nurses' hand lotions[29]. A study by Maki *et al.*[70] suggests that there is a risk of contamination of in-use fluid by organisms from unrelated peripheral infections. Miller and Grogan exhaustively cultured patients' TPN fluids serially, they found certain patient's systems were repeatedly positive, and others always negative[81,82].

Manual contact with the infusion by medical personnel is probably the major mode by which microorganisms enter in-use fluid. *The importance of frequent and vigorous hand washing by physicians and nurses cannot be overemphasized.* The tubing should be kept as far removed as possible from reservoirs of microorganisms such as open tracheostomies, draining wounds or Foley catheters.

7.3.5 Central admixture programmes

Although two comparative studies have shown little difference in the contamination rates of fluid admixtures prepared in a central pharmacy as compared with solutions made up by nurses on the patient care unit[86,87], preparation and compounding of parenteral solutions is probably best done in a central pharmacy. Culture surveys of pharmacy-prepared solutions, before distribution to the patient care unit (Table 7.10), have found rates of contamination quite comparable with surveys of in-use fluid (Table 7.6). However, fewer Gram-negative bacilli are recovered from pharmacy-prepared solutions. Availability of laminar flow hoods to eliminate airborne contaminants is often propounded as a major advantage of central pharmacy admixture programmes. However, touch contamination is probably a greater source of extrinsic contamination of fluid and the major advantage of the central pharmacy as regards asepsis may be its physical separation from the numerous reservoirs of Gram-negative bacilli present on the ward.

There is the very real concern that a break in asepsis in the pharmacy could expose a large number of patients to contaminated products and the delay between compounding and use provides opportunity for multiplication of any introduced microorganisms. With proliferation of central pharmacy admixture programmes, in the United States, occasional common source outbreaks can be anticipated (Table 7.4). In March 1976, seven paediatric patients in a US hospital developed *E. aerogenes* septicaemia traced to contaminated 5% dextrose in 0·2% normal saline to which potassium chloride had been added in a central pharmacy[37a]. The pharmacists' technique involved using a single syringe and needle to add potassium to each eight consecutive units of fluid. The initial reservoir of *Enterobacter* was not determined. *The necessity for the most stringent attention to asepsis in central admixture programmes cannot be overemphasized.* As noted previously, *as soon as a unit has been broken, the fluid should be used promptly or refrigerated.*

If established guidelines for asepsis are rigorously followed, the hazard of common source contamination is probably outweighted by the more uniform standard of asepsis, improved quality control and particularly markedly reduced drug incompatibilities and medication errors attainable with central admixture programmes. Recognizing these advantages, the US National Coordinating Committee on Large Volume Parenterals has recently formally recommended[111] that except in medical emergencies all parenteral admixtures be prepared by pharmacists in a central designated area of the hospital.

7.3.6 In-line microbial filters

In-line membrane filters are being widely advocated to reduce the risk of sepsis from contaminated fluid and to protect patients from air embolism and particulate matter. It is recommended that filters be placed terminally, between the administration set and the cannula. The author recently reviewed the role of filters in infusion therapy[112]; a summary is contained below.

In theory filters appear to be an effective means of protection against contaminated fluid. Primarily $0 \cdot 22$- and $0 \cdot 45$-micron pore size are used for infusion therapy. The $0 \cdot 45$-micron filter prevents the passage of fungi and most bacteria although *Pseudomonas sp.*, *Esch. coli* and other Gram-negative bacilli begin to pass through the filter within 6 hours of continuous use[112], the $0 \cdot 22$-micron size blocks all bacteria and fungi[112a]. Filters, particularly the $0 \cdot 22$-micron size, significantly impede the rate of flow and readily become blocked, especially when used for periods longer than 24 hours or if air bubbles get into the line. With highly viscous solutions such as those for total parenteral nutrition, infusion pumps are usually necessary to ensure continuous flow. Recent advances in design have expanded the filter area and are able to vent air bubbles from the system but the new filters will probably be quite expensive.

Filters should reduce the hazard of infection arising from contamination during manufacture and reduce the risk of infection from contaminants introduced above the filter in the course of therapy, but obviously have no effect on organisms gaining access to fluid at points below the filter and do not prevent the passage of endotoxin. Although promising on a theoretical basis, no controlled studies have been reported in a sufficiently large population to assess their efficacy in prevention of septicaemia. The manual manipulation of the delivery system needed to install the filter for use provides one more opportunity for extrinsic contamination. Miller and Grogan found the rate of in-use contamination of fluid increased 10% with each additional filter that was placed into the system (one filter, $23 \cdot 9\%$, two, $30 \cdot 8\%$, and three, $41 \cdot 6\%$)[82].

Most disconcerting is the tendency of filters to become blocked, as this usually leads to added manipulations of the cannula and delivery system in an attempt to identify the cause of malfunction. Freeman *et al.*, in a recent uncontrolled study, found a four-fold increase in the risk of sepsis in patients receiving total parenteral nutrition through in-line filters as compared to a group in which filters were not used[113]. The marked increase in the incidence of infection in the filter group was attributed to the increased number of manipulations of the infusion system, including the catheter, by ward personnel when filters became blocked. Other investigators have suspected filters paradoxically may increase the hazard of infection in TPN for similar reasons[80,107]. Several institutions with very low rates of infection in TPN therapy do not utilize filters[80,98,107,114,114a]. A recent small controlled study in Great Britain found no differences in infusion phlebitis or infection in patients receiving conventional intravenous therapy with or without filters[75]. A final consideration is the fact that filters are expensive, costing from $0·50 to $1·50 per patient so that if they are used routinely the cost of infusion therapy is substantially increased.

In summary, in-line filters show promise for reducing the hazard of contaminated fluid. However, clinical trials to determine their efficacy in preventing infusion-related infection and to demonstrate a cost-benefit are needed before they can be recommended for routine use. Replacement of all delivery apparatus every 24–48 hours probably provides equivalent protection against infection caused by contaminated fluids. Filters may ultimately prove to be of greater value in removing potentially hazardous particulate matter[115] and in reducing infusion phlebitis[116,117].

7.4 INFECTIONS IN TOTAL PARENTERAL NUTRITION

In 1968 Dudrick, Wilmore, Vars and Rhoades reported that positive nitrogen balance could be maintained by a totally parenteral route of alimentation with hypertonic glucose solutions and protein hydrolysates[118]. In the past five years TPN has proved to be highly effective and often life-saving for patients with severe and prolonged, but reversible, gastrointestinal dysfunction.

Because solutions used in TPN are highly irritating to veins, cannulation of the central circulation is required, usually by percutaneous puncture of the subclavian or internal jugular vein. Thus, catheters must remain in the same location for prolonged periods, ranging from weeks to months. Moreover, patients requiring TPN are by definition usually very debilitated and malnourished and up to 84% have active peripheral infections[97,98,114,114a]. A considerable hazard from TPN-related infection might be anticipated.

In the early years of this new therapy, from 1969 to 1973, a number of centres reported alarmingly high rates of septicaemia complicating TPN, reaching 27% in several hospitals and averaging 7% in a nationwide survey of major centres[119] (Table 7.11). Organisms associated with infections in conventional intravenous therapy including *Staph. aureus*, enterococcus and Gram-negative bacilli were frequently implicated, but approximately 50% of septicaemias were caused by *Candida albicans*, many of which were fatal. Investigation revealed that most of the centres with high rates of infection had no uniform standards for catheter care, preparation of solutions, or administration of TPN. Solutions were administered and in many instances were prepared by a variable population

TABLE 7.11   Selected reports of septicaemia complicating total parenteral
nutrition*

			Rate of septicaemia (%)	
Senior author*	Year	Number patients	All pathogens	Candida
Wilmore	1969	25	0	0
Dudrick	1969	47	6	4
McGovern	1970	25	12	4
Aschcroft		22	22	22
Curry	1971	49	27	16
Filler	1972	134	15	17
Parsa	1972	307	9	2
Ryan[97]	1972	355†	7	3
Freeman	1972	111	7	7
CDC—US Survey	1973	2078	7	4
Dillon	1973	122	4	2
Sanderson	1973	100	1	0
Copeland[114a]	1974	93	2	2
Abel[123]	1974	64	0	0

* Except for three cited instances, from studies reviewed in Maki et al.[8]
† Number of catheters

of ward personnel. Blood products were frequently given through the
TPN catheter and the line was often used to monitor central venous
pressure and draw blood[120].

Reasons for the extraordinary predominance of *Candida* in TPN-
related sepsis are conjectural and have been explored in previous communi-
cations[8,119]. Besides host factors, the nature of the solutions themselves
may be of considerable importance. *Candida* grows rapidly in many of
these protein hydrolysate–dextrose solutions, often faster than most
common bacterial pathogens[121] (and see Chapter 2). However, there
is little evidence that fluid contaminated by *Candida* causes candida
septicaemias in TPN. With only one exception[73], *Candida* has been a
rare contaminant in TPN solutions, whether sampled immediately after
preparation in the pharmacy (Table 7.10) or during administration to
patients (Table 7.9) and candida septicaemia associated with contaminated infusate has been rare[82,107,108]. Most sepsis in TPN, particularly with *Candida*, originates from the catheter. The TPN solutions
probably create a local milieu in the catheter thrombus which is selectively

advantageous to *Candida*. With a programme of rigorous site care, Sanderson and Deitel were able to administer TPN without the use of in-line filters with no candidaemia and only one bacteraemia in 100 courses of therapy[80].

Recent reports from a number of centres with such programmes have demonstrated convincingly that TPN can be delivered with minimal complications through the same catheter for prolonged periods even in extremely debilitated patients, many with active infections[97,98,114,114a], or even neutropaenia[98]. Rates of TPN-related septicaemia can be kept to less than 5% and in some centres essentially to zero[122,123] (Table 7.11). This standard of care and degree of success with rare exception requires a team to care for the infusion. Freeman, *et al.*[107] found that TPN infusions cared for by a team had a nine-fold lower incidence of septic complications ($2 \cdot 3\%$) as compared to infusions attended by ward personnel ($21 \cdot 2\%$). *A highly organized, strict protocol approach to management of infusions for TPN, which particularly emphasizes meticulous care of the catheter site, is imperative for the safe administration of TPN therapy.* Detailed guidelines for aseptic administration of TPN have been published by Goldmann and the author[119].

7.5 INTRAVENOUS THERAPY TEAMS

Because a team approach has markedly reduced the incidence of infections in TPN, intravenous therapy teams made up of nurses or technicians trained in cannula insertion and care are being widely advocated in the USA as the most effective means of administering conventional infusion therapy[8,124-126]. Although controlled clinical studies are not yet available, it is very unlikely that the very heterogenous population of medical students, house officers, physicians and nurses who usually participate in the administration of infusion therapy, particularly in large hospitals, can provide the uniform and high quality of asepsis possible with a specially trained team following a specific protocol[124]. The existence of a team permits all infusions in the hospital to be evaluated at least daily, ensuring a greater use of steel needles in preference to plastic catheters, a more reliable 48-hour catheter change, earlier removal in the presence of malfunction, inflammation or suspected infection, a more prompt recognition and treatment of infusion-related septicaemia, an earlier detection of epidemic problems, an evaluation of new infection control measures by controlled clinical trial, and a continuous resource for education of all medical personnel involved in administration of infusion therapy.

7.6 DETECTION OF EXTRINSIC CONTAMINATION AND GENERAL MANAGEMENT OF RELATED SEPSIS

Methods for detection of contamination of infusion fluid have been discussed in Chapter 2. There are three major ways to detect extrinsic contamination of the infusion, by recognition of related clinical illness, by surveillance and by quality control microbiological sampling.

7.6.1 Identification of clinical illness

Although the most stringent programme of asepsis in administration of infusion therapy will reduce substantially the incidence of related septicaemia, sporadic cases and occasional outbreaks due to extrinsic contamination and rarely intrinsic contamination will continue to occur. A favourable outcome in a given case and detection of an epidemic are heavily dependant upon recognizing the causal relationship of infusion therapy to a given case of septicaemia. The general clinical features of infusion-related septicaemia are indistinguishable from blood stream infection arising from other sites such as the urinary tract or surgical wounds[4,8,127] (Table 7.12). In particular, we have found in a recent study that catheter-related sepsis in an intensive care unit population can be extraordinarily insidious[128]. Often it is attributed to pneumonia, urinary tract or surgical wound infection, or is considered cryptogenic and treated empirically.

Several features are commonly present and point strongly towards the infusion as a cause of sepsis (Table 7.12)[4,8,129]. These are phlebitis,

TABLE 7.12   Clinical features of infusion-related septicaemia

Non-specific	Suggestive of infusion-related aetiology
Fever	Phlebitis (50%)
Chills, shaking rigors	Source of sepsis inapparent
Hypotension, shock	Patient unlikely candidate for sepsis
Hyperventilation	(i.e., young or no underlying diseases)
Gastrointestinal	
Abdominal pain	Abrupt onset, associated with shock
Vomiting	Sepsis refractory to antimicrobial therapy
Diarrhoea	or dramatic improvement with removal
Neurological	of cannula and infusion
Confusion	
Seizures	

(present in about one-half of cases), the fact that the patient is an unlikely candidate for septicaemia (for instance, he may be young or without underlying predisposing factors), or that there is no identifiable source of the septicaemia, or that sepsis may be abrupt and disproportionately severe, associated with frank shock such as was observed in the British Devonport[6] and US Cutter[7] incidents, or as is common in suppurative phlebitis[48,49], or, most characteristically, sepsis is refractory to antimicrobial therapy until the offending infusion has been removed.

When infusion-related septicaemia is suspected, blood cultures should be obtained from two separate sites of venepuncture and the entire infusion must be removed. Remaining infusate should be cultured (see Chapter 2) as well as the cannula (preferably by the SQ technique). Further recommendations for therapy have been published[8,129].

Overwhelming sepsis is relatively uncommon in uncomplicated cannula-related infection and strongly suggests venous suppuration or a massively contaminated infusate. In burn patients, local signs of inflammation at the catheter site are commonly absent with suppurative phlebitis[48,49]. Severe, unremitting septicaemia is the usual manifestation, commonly presenting from 2–10 days after catheter removal. Many cases are discovered only at autopsy. Milking the vein from above toward the puncture wound at the bedside may express pus which strongly suggests the diagnosis and should be done routinely whenever a venous cannula is removed[45]. However, if this manoeuvre does not reveal the diagnosis, but the entity is suspected, exploratory venotomy is indicated. *The most important aspect of therapy of suppurative phlebitis is surgical exclusion by resection or ligation of the involved venous segment.*

7.6.2 Surveillance

7.6.2.1 *Of infusions*

Many centres with a very low incidence of infections in TPN and in conventional intravenous therapy see each patient every 24–48 hours, routinely undressing the site, scrubbing it with antiseptics and reapplying topical antimicrobial ointment. Such a rigorous programme of care is not feasible in most hospitals without an intravenous therapy team and may not be necessary, but surveillance can still be achieved. *Each patient should be seen daily by a ward nurse and specifically queried regarding pain or tenderness at the infusion site; the presence of fever, chills or other signs of infection should be sought.* If desired, the site can be inspected and ointment reapplied every other day. *If unexplained fever, local inflammation or purulence are noted, the cannula and entire infusion must immediately be removed.* However, it is important to realize that cannulae can cause septicaemia in the absence of local inflammation.

7.6.2.2   Of clinical infections

Surveillance of all bacteraemic infections and in particular of primary bacteraemias (those without a clinically apparent source) can identify contamination leading to illness, particularly occurring on an epidemic scale in the hospital[4] or nationally[4,130,131] (and see Chapter 2). However, it has not been established and is controversial if routine clinical surveillance of *all* nosocomial infection is justifiable on a cost-benefit basis[132].

TABLE 7.13   **Microbial pathogens associated with infusion-related septicaemia**

Source of septicaemia	Major pathogens
Conventional intravenous therapy	
Cannula	Staph. aureus (approx. 50%)
	Klebsiella–Enterobacter
	Serratia
	enterococcus
	Ps. aeruginosa
	Ps. cepacia
Contaminated fluid	Tribe Klebsielleae (90%)
	Klebsiella
	Enterobacter*
	Serratia
	Ps. cepacia*
	Citrobacter freundii
Total Parenteral Nutrition	Candida spp. (50%)
	Torulopsis glabrata
	Staph. aureus
	Klebsiella–Enterobacter
	enterococcus
Contaminated blood products	Pseudomonads
	Achromobacter
	Citrobacter
	Flavobacterium
Related to arterial catheter-pressure monitoring catheters	Ps. cepacia*
	Enterobacter*
	Flavobacterium

* In particular, septicaemia caused by *E. cloacae* or especially *E. agglomerans* or *Ps. cepacia* should prompt search for contaminated infusion fluid

7.6.2.3 *Microbiological*

The microbiological profile of infusion-related septicaemia (Table 7.13) is sufficiently characteristic to be of considerable value in detection of extrinsic contamination, particularly septicaemia related to TPN and to contaminated infusate (Chapter 2). *But, for microbiological surveillance to be maximially effective, all blood isolates must be routinely speciated.* In 1970–71, a number of US hospitals without clinical surveillance programmes, and who also did not routinely fully characterize all blood isolates, experienced significant epidemics of infusion-related septicaemia that were recognized only in retrospect[4].

Cryptogenic staphylococcal bacteraemia, candidaemia in a patient receiving TPN, and all bacteraemias caused by tribe Klebsielleae organisms (especially *E. agglomerans*) and *Ps. cepacia* in the setting of infusion therapy must prompt search for an infusion-related aetiology. Epidemic clusters of bacteraemic infection with any organism, but particularly those in Table 7.13 warrant intensive investigation.

If intrinsic contamination is suspected, that is, there has been proven contamination of infusion fluid or a cluster of infusion-related septicaemias, pertinent data including the lot numbers of suspected products should immediately be transmitted to appropriate local and national public health authorities. Remaining products should be retained for their evaluation.

7.6.3. Quality control microbiological sampling

7.6.3.1 *Infusion fluid*

Although a number of hospitals in the US now carry out routine micro-biological sampling of fluid admixtures[78, 93–95] either after pharmacy compounding or in-use, the cost-benefit of such programmes is unknown (Chapter 2). There is probably much more yield in routinely sampling fluids of patients with clinical signs of sepsis or who are specifically suspected of suffering from infusion-related infection.

Data was presented in Chapter 2 to suggest that an outbreak due to intrinsically contaminated products of the magnitude that Abbott experienced in 1970–71 might conceivably have been detected by current US intrahospital programmes of quality control microbiological sampling of fluid.

7.6.3.2 *Cannulae*

Because cannula-related infection is much more common, and is clinically more insidious, a programme of culturing vascular cannulae on removal is less controversial and far more likely to provide useful data. Certain cannulae should routinely be cultured, including all plastic catheters removed from high-risk patients, particularly burn patients or patients receiving TPN, catheters associated with phlebitis, and certainly all cannulae (both catheters and needles) from patients with clinically suspected infusion-related sepsis. The SQ culture method described earlier[21] can provide useful data.

A hospital may elect periodically to culture all catheters (or cannulae) to obtain baseline information pertaining to the existing level of asepsis in catheter (cannula) care. Such programmes can be utilized to evaluate critically new infection control measures such as the use of topical anti-microbial agents, or even an intravenous therapy team.

Acknowledgements

I acknowledge the contribution of a prior close professional association with Frank S. Rhame, MD (Stanford Veteran's Hospital, Palo Alto, California) and Donald A. Goldmann, MD (Children's Hospital Medical Center, Boston, Massachusetts), friends and former colleagues at the US Center for Disease Control, to the formulation of many concepts contained in this chapter.

References

1. Center for Disease Control. (1971). Nosocomial bacteremias associated with intravenous fluid therapy—USA. *Morbid. Mortal. Weekly Rep.*, **20** (Suppl.)
2. Felts, S. K., Shaffner, W., Melly, M. A. and Koenig, M. G. (1972). Sepsis caused by contaminated intravenous fluids: epidemiologic, clinical and laboratory investigations of an outbreak in one hospital. *Ann. Intern. Med.*, **77**, 881
3. Fisher, E. J., Maki, D. G., Eisses, J. and Quinn, E. (1971). Epidemic septicemias due to intrinsically contaminated infusion products. Abstracts of papers presented at the *Eleventh Interscience Conference for Anti-microbial Agents and Chemotherapy*. October 20, Atlantic City
4. Maki, D. G., Rhame, F. S., Mackel, D. C. and Bennett, J. V. (1976). Nationwide epidemic of septicemia caused by contaminated intravenous products: epidemiologic and clinical features. *Am. J. Med.*, **60**, 471
5. Phillips, I., Eykyn, S. and Laker, M. (1972). Outbreak of hospital infection caused by contaminated autoclaved fluids. *Lancet*, **i**, 1258
6. Meers, P. D., Calder, M. W., Mazhar, M. M. and Lawrie, G. M. (1973). Intravenous infusion of contaminated dextrose solution. *Lancet*, **ii**, 1189

7. Center for Disease Control. (1973). Septicemias associated with contaminated intravenous fluids. *Morbid. Mortal. Weekly Rep.*, **22**, 99

8. Maki, D. G., Goldmann, D. A. and Rhame, F. S. (1973). Infection control in intravenous therapy. *Ann. Intern. Med.*, **79**, 867

9. Druskin, M. S. and Siegel, P. D. (1963). Bacterial contamination of indwelling intravenous polyethylene catheters. *J. Am. Med. Ass.*, **185**, 966

10. Moran, J. M., Atwood, R. P. and Rowe, M. I. (1965). A clinical and bacteriologic study of infections associated with venous cut-downs. *N. Engl. J. Med.*, **272**, 554

11. Smits, H. and Freedman, I. R. (1967). Prolonged venous catheterization as a cause of sepsis. *N. Engl. J. Med.*, **276**, 1229

12. Bernard, R. W., Stahl, W. M. and Chase, R. M. (1971). Subclavian vein catheterizations: A prospective study. II. Infectious complications. *Ann. Surg.*, **173**, 191

13. Henzel, J. H. and DeWeese, M. S. (1971). Morbid and mortal complications associated with prolonged central venous cannulation. *Am. J. Surg.*, **121**, 600

14. Mogensen, J. V., Frederiksen, W. and Jensen, J. K. (1972). Subclavian vein catheterization and infection: A bacteriologic study of 130 catheter insertions. *Scand. J. Infect. Dis.*, **4**, 31

15. Colvin, M. P., Blogg, C. E., Savege, T. M. *et al.* (1972). A safe long-term infusion technique? *Lancet*, **ii**, 317

16. Hoshal, V. L. (1972). Intravenous catheters and infection. *Surg. Clin. N. Am.*, **52**, 1407

17. Francke, D. E. (editor). (1970). *Handbook of IV Additive Reviews*, p. 18 (Hamilton, Illinois: Hamilton Press)

18. Hoshal, V. L., Ause, R. G. and Hoskins, P. A. (1971). Fibrin sleeve formation on indwelling subclavian central venous catheters. *Arch. Surg.*, **102**, 253

19. Peters, W. R., Bush, W. H., McIntyre, R. D. and Hill, L. D. (1973). The development of fibrin sheath on indwelling venous catheters. *Surg. Gynecol. Obstet.*, **137**, 43

20. Turco, S. J. (1975). Phlebitis associated with intravenous drug administration. *Bull. Paren. Drug Assoc.*, **29**, 89

21. Maki, D. G., Weise, C. E. and Sarafin, H. W. (1976). Semi-quantitative method for identifying intravenous catheter-related infection. *Clin. Res.*, **24**, 25A

22. Pollack, M., Charache, P., Nieman, R. E., Jett, M. P., Reinhardt, J. A. and Hardy, P. H. Jr. (1972). Factors influencing colonization and antibiotic-resistant patterns of Gram-negative bacteria in hospital patients. *Lancet*, **ii**, 668

23. Salzman, T. C., Clark, J. J. and Klemm, L. (1968). Hand contamination of personnel as a mechanism of cross-infection in nosocomial infections with antibiotic-resistant *Escherichia coli* and *Klebsiella-Aerobacter*. *Antimicrob. Agents Chemother.*, **1967**, 97

24. Knittle, M. A., Eitzman, D. V. and Baer, J. (1975). Role of hand contamination of personnel in epidemiology of Gram-negative nosocomial infections. *J. Pediatr.*, **86**, 433

25. Brereton, R. B. (1969). Incidence of complications from indwelling venous catheters. *Del. Med. J.*, **41**, 1

26. Banks, D. C., Yates, D. B., Cawdrey, H. M. *et al.* (1970). Infection from intravenous catheters. *Lancet*, **i**, 443

27. Darrell, J. H. and Garrod, L. P. (1969). Secondary septicaemia from intravenous cannulae. *Br. Med. J.*, **2**, 481

28. Roberts, R. J. and Cockcroft, W. H. (1970). Infection associated with intravenous catheters. *Can. Med. Ass. J.*, **102**, 89

29. Morse, L. J., Williams, H. L., Grenn, F. P. *et al.* (1967). Septicemia due to *Klebsiella pneumoniae* originating from a hand cream dispenser. *N. Engl. J. Med.*, **277**, 472

29a. Lowbury, E. J. L., Lilly, H. A. and Bull, J. P. (1964). Methods for disinfection of hands and operation sites. *Br. Med. J.*, **2**, 531

29b. White, J. J., Wallace, C. K. and Burnett, L. S. (1970). Skin disinfection. *Johns Hopkins Med. J.*, **126**, 169

30. Plotkin, S. A. and Austrian, R. (1958). Bacteremia caused by *Pseudomonas* sp. following the use of materials stored in solutions of a cationic surface-active agent. *Am. J. Med. Sci.*, **235**, 621

31. Malizia, W. F., Gangarosa, E. J. and Goley, A. F. (1960). Benzalkonium chloride as a source of infection. *N. Engl. J. Med.*, **263**, 800

32. Sack, R. A. (1970). Epidemic of Gram-negative organism septicemia subsequent to elective operation. *Am. J. Obstet. Gynecol.*, **107**, 394

33. Phillips, I., Eykyn, S., Curtis, M. A. and Snell, J. J. S. (1971). *Pseudomonas cepacia* (multivorans) septicemia in an intensive care unit. *Lancet*, **i**, 375

34. Speller, D. C. E., Stephens, M. E. and Viant, A. C. (1971). Hospital infection by *Pseudomonas cepacia*. *Lancet*, **i**, 798

35. Stamm, W. E., Colella, J. J., Anderson, R. L. and Dixon, R. E. (1975). Indwelling arterial catheters as a source of nosocomial bacteremia. *N. Engl. J. Med.*, **292**, 1099

36. Center for Disease Control. (1974). Nosocomial *Pseudomonas cepacia* bacteremia caused by contaminated pressure transducers. *Morbid. Mortal. Weekly Rep.*, **23**, 423

37. Center for Disease Control. (1975). Transducer-associated bacteremia. *Morbid. Mortal. Weekly Rep.*, **24**, 295

37a. Primary Bacteremia—Illinois. (1976). *Morbid. Mortal. Weekly Rep.*, **25**, 110

38. Lee, J. C. and Fiaklow, P. J. (1961). Benzalkonium chloride—source of hospital infection with Gram-negative bacteria. *J. Am. Med. Ass.*, **177**, 708

38a. Bassett, D. C. J. (1971). The effect of pH on the multiplication of a pseudomonad in chlorhexidine and cetrimide. *J. Clin. Pathol.*, **24**, 708

39. Lowenbraun, S., Young, V., Kenton, D., *et al.* (1970). Infection from intravenous 'scalp-vein' needles in a susceptible population. *J. Am. Med. Ass.*, **212**, 451

40. Peter, G., Lloyd-Still, J. D. and Lovejoy, F. H. (1972). Local infection and bacteremia from scalp vein needles and polyethylene catheters in children. *J. Pediatr.*, **80**, 78

41. Crossley, K. and Matsen, J. M. (1972). The scalp vein needle: A prospective study of associated complications. *J. Am. Med. Ass.*, **220**, 985

42. Crenshaw, C. A., Kelly, L., Turner, R. J. *et al.* (1972). Prevention of infection at scalp vein sites of needles insertion during intravenous therapy. *Am. J. Surg.*, **124**, 43

43. Keogh, E. J. and Hopkins, B. E. (1973). Risk of infection with scalp vein needles—A prospective study. *Aust. N.Z. J. Med.*, **3**, 389
44. Harbin, R. L. and Schaffner, W. (1973). Septicemia associated with scalp-vein needles. *South. Med. J.*, **66**, 638
45. Maki, D. G., Drinka, P. J. and Davis, T. E. (1975). Suppurative phlebitis of an arm vein from a 'scalp-vein needle'. *N. Engl. J. Med.*, **292**, 1116
46. Crane, C. (1960). Venous interruption for septic thrombophlebitis. *N. Engl. J. Med.*, **262**, 947
47. Foley, F. D. (1969). The burn autopsy: fatal complication of burns. *Am. J. Clin. Pathol.*, **52**, 1
48. Pruitt, B. A., Stein, J. M. and Foley, F. D. (1970). Intravenous therapy in burn patients—suppurative thrombophlebitis and other life-threatening complications. *Arch. Surg.*, **100**, 399
49. Stein, J. M. and Pruitt, B. A. (1970). Suppurative thrombophlebitis—a lethal iatrogenic disease. *N. Engl. J. Med.*, **282**, 1452
50. Barenholtz, L., Kaminsky, N. I. and Palmer, D. L. (1973). Venous intramural microabscess. A cause of protracted sepsis with intravenous cannulas. *Am. J. Med. Sci.*, **365**, 335
51. Warden, G. D., Wilmore, D. W. and Pruitt, B. A. (1973). Central venous thrombosis: A hazard of medical progress. *J. Trauma*, **13**, 620
52. Cormier, M. and Lecompte, Y. (1973). Ligation of veins in suppurative thrombophlebitis secondary to venous catheterization. *Surg. Gynecol. Obstet.*, **138**, 662
53. Munster, A. M. (1974). Septic thrombophlebitis. A surgical disorder. *J. Am. Med. Ass.*, **230**, 1010
54. Popp, M. G., Law, E. J. and MacMillan, B. G. (1974). Parenteral nutrition in the burned child: A study of twenty-six patients. *Ann. Surg.*, **179**, 219
55. Maki, D. G. and Jarrett, F. (1976). Semi-quantitative culture method for identifying vascular catheter-related septicemia in the burn patient. *Surg. Forum* (submitted for publication)
56. Zinner, S. H., Denny-Brown, B. C., Braun, P. *et al.* (1969). Risk of infection with intravenous indwelling catheters: effect of application of antibiotic ointment. *J. Infect. Dis.*, **120**, 616
57. Norden, C. W. (1969). Application of antibiotic ointment to the site of venous catheterization—a controlled trial. *J. Infect. Dis.*, **120**, 611
58. Levy, R. S., Goldstein, J. and Pressman, R. S. (1970). Value of a topical antibiotic ointment in reducing bacterial colonization of percutaneous venous catheters. *J. Albert Einstein Med. Ctr.*, **18**, 67
59. Crenshaw, C. A., Kelly, L., Turner, R. J. *et al.* (1972). Bacteriologic nature and prevention of contamination to intravenous catheters. *Am. J. Surg.*, **123**, 264
60. Irwin, G. R., Hart, R. K. and Martin, C. M. (1973). Pathogenesis and prevention of intravenous catheter infections. *Yale J. Biol. Med.*, **46**, 85
61. Michaelson, E. D. and Walsh, R. E. (1970). Osler's node—a complication of prolonged arterial cannulation. *N. Engl. J. Med.*, **283**, 472
62. Gardner, R. M., Schwartz, R., Wong, H. C. and Burke, J. P. (1974). Percutaneous indwelling radial-artery catheters for monitoring cardiovascular function. Prospective study of the risk of thrombosis and infection. *N. Engl. J. Med.*, **290**, 1227

63. Bedford, R. F. and Wollman, H. (1973). Complications of percutaneous radial-artery cannulation: An objective prospective study in man. *Anesthetics*, **38**, 228

64. Todres, I. D., Rogers, M. C., Shannon, D. C., Moylan, F. M. B. and Ryan, J. F. (1975). Percutaneous catheterization of the radial artery in the critically ill neonate. *J. Pediatr.*, **87**, 273

65. Maki, D. G. and McCormick, R. (1976). Septic endarteritis due to intra-arterial catheters for cancer chemotherapy. I. Clinical features and management. II. Investigation of an outbreak. III. Risk factors and prevention. (Submitted for publication)

66. Michaels, L. and Ruebner, B. (1953). Growth of bacteria in intravenous infusion fluids. *Lancet*, **i**, 772

67. Wilmore, D. W. and Dudrick, S. J. (1969). An in-line filter for intravenous solutions. *Arch. Surg.*, **99**, 462

68. Robertson, M. H. (1970). Fungi in fluids—a hazard of intravenous therapy. *J. Med. Microbiol.*, **3**, 99

69. Duma, R. J., Warner, J. F. and Dalton, H. P. (1971). Septicemia from intravenous infusions. *N. Engl. J. Med.*, **284**, 257

70. Maki, D. G., Anderson, R. L. and Shulman, J. A. (1974). In-use contamination of intravenous infusion fluid. *Appl. Microbiol.*, **28**, 778

71. Maki, D. G., Rhame, F. S., Goldmann, D. A. and Mandell, G. L. (1973). The infection hazard posed by contaminated intravenous infusion fluid. *Bacteremia-Laboratory and Clinical Aspects*. p. 76 (Springfield, Illinois: Charles C. Thomas)

72. Maki, D. G. and Martin, W. T. (1975). Nationwide epidemic of septicemia caused by contaminated infusion products. IV. Growth of microbial pathogens in fluids for intravenous infusion. *J. Infect. Dis.*, **131**, 267

73. Deeb, E. N. and Natsios, G. A. (1971). Contamination of intravenous fluids by bacteria and fungi during preparation and administration. *Am. J. Hosp. Pharm.*, **28**, 764

74. Letcher, K. I., Thrupp, L. D., Schapiro, D. J. *et al.* (1972). In-use contamination of intravenous solutions in flexible plastic containers. *Am. J. Hosp. Pharm.*, **29**, 673

75. Collin, J., Tweedle, D. E. F., Venables, C. W., Constable, F. L. and Johnston, I. D. A. (1973). Effect of a millipore filter on complications of intravenous infusions: A prospective clinical trial. *Br. Med. J.*, **4**, 456

76. Ernerot, L., Thoren, S. and Sandell, E. (1973). Studies on microbial contamination of infusion fluids arising from drug additions and administration. *Acta Pharm. Suecica*, **10**, 141

77. Steckel, S. D., Gonik, M., Martens, P. J., Patel, J. A., Curtis, E. G. and Ho, N. F. (1973). *Drug Intell. Clin. Pharm.*, **7**, 177

78. Ravin, R., Bahr, J. *et al.* (1974). Program for bacterial surveillance of intravenous admixtures. *Am. J. Hosp. Pharm.*, **31**, 340

78a. Woodside, W., Woodside, M. E., D'Arcy, P. F. and Patel, R. H. (1975). Intravenous fluids as vehicles of infection. *Pharm. J.*, **215**, 606

79. Asch, M. J., Huxtable, R. F. and Hays, D. M. (1972). High calorie parenteral therapy in infants and children. *Arch. Surg.*, **104**, 434

80. Sanderson, I. and Deitel, M. (1973). Intravenous hyperalimentation without sepsis. *Surg. Gynecol. Obstet.*, **136**, 577

81. Miller, R. C. and Grogan, J. B. (1975). Efficacy of in-line bacterial filters in reducing contamination of intravenous nutritional solutions. *Am. J. Surg.*, **130**, 585

82. Miller, R. C. and Grogan, J. B. (1973). Incidence and source of contamination of intravenous nutritional infusion systems. *J. Pediatr. Surg.*, **8**, 185

83. Spatz, M., Ho, N. F., Curtis, M. G. and Patel, J. A. (1973). The sterility of a screw-capped bottle system containing irrigating solutions. *Drug Intell. Clin. Pharm.*, **7**, 473

84. Carney, W. (1971). Management of intravenous infusions. *N. Engl. J. Med.*, **284**, 1037

84a. Mackel, D. C., Maki, D. G., Anderson, R. L., Rhame, F. S. and Bennett, J. V. (1975). Nationwide epidemic of septicemia caused by contaminated intravenous products: mechanisms of intrinsic contamination. *J. Clin. Microbiol.*, **2**, 486

84b. Allwood, M. C. (1975). Microbial contamination of sterile fluids in glass containers. *J. Hosp. Pharm.*, **33**, 119

85. Garvan, J. M. and Gunner, B. W., (1964). The harmful effects of particles in intravenous fluids. *Med. J. Aust.*, **2**, 1

86. Miller, W. A., Smith, G. L. and Latiolais, C. J. (1971). A comparative evaluation of compounding costs and contamination rates of intravenous admixture systems. *Drug Intell. Clin. Pharm.*, **5**, 51

87. Poretz, D. M., Guynn, J. B., Duma, R. J. and Dalton, H. P. (1974). Microbial contamination of glass bottle (open-vented) and plastic bag (closed-nonvented) intravenous fluid delivery systems. *Am. J. Hosp. Pharm.*, **31**, 726

88. McAllister, J. C., Buchanan, E. C. and Skolaut, M. W. (1974). A comparison of the safety and efficiency of three intermittent intravenous therapy systems—the minibottle, the minibag and the in-line burette. *Am. J. Hosp. Pharm.*, **31**, 961

89. Perceval, A. K. (1966). Contamination of parenteral solutions during administration. *Med. J. Aust.*, **2**, 954

90. Arnold, T. R. and Hepler, C. D. (1971). Bacterial contamination of intravenous fluids opened in unsterile air. *Am. J. Hosp. Pharm.*, **28**, 614

91. Hansen, J. S. and Hepler, C. D. (1973). Contamination of intravenous solutions by airborne microbes. *Am. J. Hosp. Pharm.*, **30**, 326

92. Greene, V. W., Vesley, D., Bond, R. G. and Michaelsen, G. S. (1962). Microbiological contamination of hospital air. II. Qualitative studies.

93. Buth, J. A., Coverly, R. W. and Eckel, F. M. (1973). A practical method of sterility monitoring of IV admixtures and a method of implementing a routine sterility monitoring program. *Drug Intell. Clin. Pharm.*, **7**, 276

94. Kundsin, R. B., Walter, C. W. and Scott, J. A. (1973). In-use testing of sterility of intravenous solutions in plastic containers. *Surgery*, **73**, 778

95. Hanson, A. L. and Shelley, R. M. (1974). Monitoring contamination levels of intravenous solutions using 'total-sample' techniques. *Am. J. Hosp. Pharm.*, **31**, 733

96. Hak, L. J., Long, J. M., Ruberg, R. L. *et al.* (1971). Contamination incidence in IV solutions with additives. Presented to the Annual Meeting of the American Society of Hospital Pharmacists, 31 March 1971

97. Ryan, J. A., Abel, R. M., Abbott, W. M. *et al.* (1974). Catheter complications in total parenteral nutrition: A prospective study of 200 consecutive patients. *N. Engl. J. Med.*, **290**, 757
98. Copeland, E. M., MacFadyen, B. V. and Dudrick, S. J. (1974). Prevention of microbial catheter contamination in patients receiving parenteral hyperalimentation. *South. Med. J.*, **67**, 303
99. Herman, L. G. (1970). A critical evaluation of microbiological hazards associated with the pharmacy and the hospital. *Am. J. Hosp. Pharm.*, **27**, 56
100. D'Arcy, P. F. and Woodside, W. (1973). Drug additives: A potential source of bacterial contamination of infusion fluids. *Lancet*, **ii**, 96
101. McArthur, B. J., Hargiss, C. and Schoenknecht, F. D. (1975). Stopcock contamination in an ICU. *Am. J. Nursing*, **75**, 96
102. James, J. D. (1959). Bacterial contamination of reserved blood. *Vox Sang.*, **4**, 177
103. Buchholz, D. H., Young, V. M., Friedman, N. R. *et al.* (1971). Bacterial proliferation in platelet products stored at room temperature. *N. Engl. J. Med.*, **285**, 429
104. Stevens, A. R., Legg, J. S., Henry, B. S. *et al.* (1953). Fatal transfusion reactions from contamination of stored blood by cold growing bacteria. *Ann. Intern. Med.*, **39**, 1228
105. Braude, A. I. (1958). Transfusion reactions from contaminated blood. Their recognition and treatment. *N. Engl. J. Med.*, **258**, 1289
106. Rhame, F. S., Root, F. K., MacLowry, T. A. *et al.* (1973). Salmonella septicemia from platelet transfusions. *Ann. Intern. Med.*, **78**, 633
107. Freeman, J. B., Lemire, A. and MacLean, L. D. (1972). Intravenous alimentation and septicemia. *Surg. Gynecol. Obstet.*, **135**, 708
108. Boeckman, C. R. and Krill, C. E. Jr. (1970). Bacterial and fungal infections complicating parenteral alimentation in infants and children. *J. Pediatr. Surg.*, **5**, 117
109. Weyrauch, H. M. and Bassett, J. B. (1951). Ascending infection in an artificial urinary tract; an experimental study. *Stanford Med. Bull.*, **9**, 25
110. Ashcraft, K. W. and Leape, L. L. (1970). Candida sepsis complicating parenteral feeding. *J. Am. Med. Ass.*, **212**, 454
111. US National Coordinating Committee on Large Volume Parenterals. (1975). Recommended system for surveillance and reporting of problems with large-volume parenterals in hospitals. *Am. J. Hosp. Pharm.*, **32**, 1251
112a. Rusmin, S., Althauser, M. B. and DeLuca, P. P. (1975). Consequence of microbial contamination during extended intravenous therapy using in-line filters. *Am. J. Hosp. Pharm.*, **32**, 373
112. Maki, D. G. (1976). Final Filters. *Hosp. Inf. Control*, **3**, 22
113. Feeman, J. B. and Litton, A. A. (1974). Preponderance of Gram-positive infections during parenteral alimentation. *Surg. Gynecol. Obstet.*, **139**, 905
114. Dillon, J. D., Schaffner, W., Van Way, C. W. and Meng, H. C. (1973). Septicemia and total parenteral nutrition. Distinguishing catheter-related from other septic episodes. *J. Am. Med. Ass.*, **223**, 1341
114a. Copeland, E. M., MacFadyen, B. V., McGown, C. and Dudrick, S. J. (1974). The use of hyperalimentation in patients with potential sepsis. *Surg. Gynecol. Obstet.*, **138**, 377

115. Turco, S. and Davis, N. M. (1973). Clinical significance of particulate matter; a review of the literature. *Hosp. Pharm.*, **8**, 137

116. Ryan, P. B., Rapp, R. P., DeLuca, P. O. *et al.* (1973). In-line final filtration —a method of minimizing the risk of bacterial, fungal, and particle contamination in intravenous therapy. *Bull. Parenter. Drug Ass.*, **27**, 1

117. DeLuca, P. O., Rapp, R. P., Bivins, B., McKean, H. E. and Griffen, W. O. (1975). Filtration and infusion phlebitis: a double-blind prospective study. *Am. J. Hosp. Pharm.*, **32**, 1001

118. Dudrick, S. J., Wilmore, D. W., Vars, H. M. *et al.* (1968). Long-term total parenteral nutrition with growth, development, and positive nitrogen balance. *Surgery*, **64**, 134

119. Goldmann, D. A. and Maki, D. G. (1973). Infection control in total parenteral nutrition. *J. Am. Med. Ass.*, **223**, 1360

120. Curry, C. R. and Quie, P. G. (1971). Fungal septicemia in patients receiving parenteral hyperalimentation. *N. Engl. J. Med.*, **285**, 1221

121. Goldmann, D. A., Martin, W. T. and Worthington, J. W. (1973). Growth of bacteria and fungi in total parenteral nutrition solutions. *Am. J. Surg.*, **126**, 314

122. Wilmore, D. W. and Dudrick, S. J. (1969). Safe long-term venous catheterization. *Arch. Surg.*, **98**, 256

123. Abel, R. M., Fischer, J. E., Buckley, M. J. and Austen, W. G. (1974). Hyperalimentation in cardiac surgery; a review of sixty-four patients. *Surg. Gynecol. Obstet.*, **139**, 468

124. Bentley, D. E. and Lepper, M. H. (1968). Septicemia related to indwelling venous catheter. *J. Am. Med. Ass.*, **206**, 1749

125. Corso, J. A., Agostinelli, R. and Brandriss, M. W. (1969). Maintenance of venous polyethylene catheters to reduce risk of infection. *J. Am. Med. Ass.*, **210**, 2075

126. Fuchs, P. C. (1971). Indwelling intravenous polyethylene catheters. Factors influencing the risk of microbial colonization and sepsis. *J. Am. Med. Ass.*, **216**, 1447

127. Freeman, R. and King, B. (1975). Recognition of infection associated with intravenous catheters. *Br. J. Surg.*, **62**, 404

128. Maki, D. G. and Agger, W. (1976). The profile of vascular catheter-related septicemia in an intensive care unit population. (In preparation for publication)

129. Maki, D. G. (1976). Preventing infection in intravenous therapy. *Hosp. Pract.*, **11**, 95

130. Bennett, J. V., Scheckler, W. E., Maki, D. G. *et al.* (1971). Current National Patterns, United States. *Proceedings of the International Conference on Nosocomial Infections.* (Chicago: American Hospital Association)

131. Goldmann, D. A., Fulkerson, C. C., Dixon, R. E., Maki, D. G. and Bennett, J. V. (1976). Nationwide epidemic of septicemias caused by contaminated intravenous products. II. Assessment of the problem by a National Nosocomial Infection Surveillance System. (Submitted for publication)

132. Cluff, L. E. (1970). Surveillance as a control system—Panel. Statement of Moderator. *Proceedings of the International Conference on Nosocomial Infections.* (Chicago: American Hospital Association)

8

Intrinsic contamination—the associated infective syndromes
R. E. Dixon

8.1 INTRODUCTION

When a contaminated therapeutic agent causes disease, no time should be lost in determining whether extrinsic or intrinsic contamination is the source. Extrinsic contamination, introduced while the product is in use often causes sporadic disease, but it also can cause major epidemics. By its nature, extrinsic contamination usually involves only a single institution. In contrast, intrinsic contamination, that is present when the product is received in the hospital, is a potentially far greater threat since medical supplies are often produced by a relatively few manufacturers, are distributed quite widely, and may, therefore, affect a large number of patients in many hospitals.

Since 1970, the Center for Disease Control (CDC) has investigated three separate epidemics of Gram-negative septicaemia caused by intrinsic contamination of fluids administered intravenously[1-4]. From the experience with these epidemics, we can (1) describe the clinical syndromes resulting from infusion of intrinsically contaminated fluids, (2) review the clues that point to epidemic bacteraemia caused by intrinsic contamination, and (3) outline an approach that should reduce the risk of such occurrences in the future.

The first epidemic, the largest of the group, began in mid-1970. Outbreaks in individual hospitals were first reported to CDC in December 1970, and they abruptly stopped when all intravenous fluids supplied by the implicated manufacturer were recalled in March 1971[1]. Dextrose-containing intravenous fluids from multiple production batches of a single manufacturer were involved. Epidemiological investigations in 25 hospitals using intravenous fluids supplied solely by that manufacturer detected 378 patients with *Enterobacter cloacae* or *Enterobacter agglomerans** bacteraemia attributed to the contaminated fluids. Organisms were introduced into the screw-cap closure after steam sterilization and apparently rarely directly contaminated the infusion fluid before clinical use. Approximately 8% of cap liners and 0·6% of unmanipulated fluids were found to contain the epidemic strains. Trauma to the caps and manipulation necessary to remove caps and set up an infusion served to inoculate fluids with microorganisms that then proliferated and caused bacteraemia. A seemingly minor change in the production process seemed to facilitate contamination. Shortly before the outbreak began, the manufacturer discontinued the use of a red rubber (Gilsonite†) cap liner and substituted in its place a synthetic (Elastomer†) liner. Gilsonite was subsequently shown to possess a diffusable substance inhibitory to the epidemic strains while Elastomer did not.

The second epidemic was recognized in 1973 in a single hospital[2,3]. It also involved multiple lots of dextrose-containing fluids—primarily 5% dextrose in lactated Ringer's solution. *Citrobacter freundii* and, again, *E. agglomerans* were the responsible pathogens. This epidemic was apparently much more limited in scope than the first, in large part because

* At the time of this outbreak, *E. agglomerans* was generally identified as *Erwinia* species, *herbicola-lathyri* group
† Trade names are provided for identification only and inclusion does not imply endorsement by the Public Health Service or the US Department of Health, Education, and Welfare

the affected hospital recognized the epidemic promptly and reported it to CDC. We know of only five cases of disease clearly related to the contaminated fluid. As in the first outbreak, available data suggest that contamination was introduced after steam-autoclave sterilization. Here, too, it is likely that a minor change in manufacturing process was responsible for the emergence of contaminated fluid. Shortly before the contaminated fluids were produced, autoclave pressures were increased; this presumably led to an excessive pressure differential between the outsides and insides of fluid containers during cooling and thereby served to draw contaminated cooling water into the fluids.

The third epidemic was unique in that it involved 25% Normal Serum Albumin rather than a dextrose-containing fluid[4]. In 1973, 11 patients in a university hospital developed *Pseudomonas* species bacteraemia statistically associated with albumin infusion. Cultures of unused fluid subsequently showed contamination with a *P. cepacia* strain compatible with the epidemic strain. Serum albumin cannot be steam autoclaved; rather it is heated at 60 °C for 10 hours and then passed through a membrane filter for sterilization. Here too, the sterilization process was not documented to be at fault; contamination seems to have been introduced after the heat treatment, probably during the subsequent filling of individual patient-use vials.

Two important features of these epidemics must be emphasized. First, in none was there documented failure of the sterilization process. Instead, contamination was probably introduced after heat sterilization. Thus, it is clear that we cannot prevent recurrences of these episodes by focusing our attention solely on sterilization procedures. Second, in at least two of the three outbreaks, relatively minor changes in the production process seem to have played a major role in allowing contamination. Neither of these changes should have been expected to produce such disastrous consequences. This emphasises how little we know about the many factors that influence the sterility of a complicated medical product.

8.2 INFECTIVE SYNDROMES

8.2.1 Clinical

Table 8.1 summarizes the clinical features seen in the three epidemics investigated by CDC. It is apparent that the clinical signs and symptoms resulting from infusion of intrinsically contaminated intravenous fluids cannot be distinguished from bacterial septicaemia arising from other sources. The incubation period between initiation of infusion and onset of

TABLE 8.1   Clinical features of epidemic cases

	Episode 1 (%)	Episode 2 (%)	Episode 3 (%)
Fever over 40 °C	53	100	36
Phlebitis	50	0	0
Hypotension	49	100	64
Improvement with treatment:			
Antibiotics only	9	0	NA
Antibiotics and discontinue infusion	95	33	NA
Discontinue infusion only	100	0	NA

NA = Not ascertainable

symptoms ranged from only a few minutes to many hours. The clinical reaction was often ushered in by a violent rigor with fever to 40 °C or even higher, but many affected patients had a more gradual temperature rise. Hypotension and other findings associated with endotoxaemia were seen in 50–100% of the patients in the various outbreaks, and other symptoms characteristic of bacterial septicaemia (gastrointestinal upset with nausea, vomiting, or diarrhoea; neurological symptoms such as delirium, hyperreactivity, or seizures) were also often noted. In the first outbreak, severe phlebitis occurred in over half of the patients within 24 hours after the start of the infusion either through steel, scalp-vein needles or plastic cannulae, but in the two other outbreaks, clinical phlebitis was not a prominent sign even though it was specifically looked for.

Two clinical features, if present, do suggest infusion bacteraemia. First, in each outbreak, dramatic clinical septicaemia was occasionally noted in patients without apparent predisposition to bacteraemia. In the second epidemic, for example, all of the infected patients in the hospital that first reported the epidemic were hospitalized for elective gynaecological surgery and none had known infection prior to onset of septicaemia. Second, the courses of the illnesses were dramatically influenced by the management of the intravenous infusions. Continued infusion of contaminated fluid led to persistence of septicaemia, even when appropriate antibiotics were given simultaneously. In contrast, discontinuation of the infusion usually produced prompt clinical improvement even when appropriate antibiotics were not given. However, it must be stressed that these characteristics are not unique to infusion of intrinsically contaminated fluids; they are also commonly seen when the infusion is contaminated extrinsically.

The clinical syndrome of infusion bacteraemia seems to be influenced by several factors. The virulence of the infecting microorganism may play some role, but even bacteria traditionally considered to have low virulence such as *E. agglomerans* and *P. cepacia* can produce fulminant and irreversible Gram-negative septicaemia when infused in large numbers. The quantity of infused microorganisms probably plays a major role in clinical outcome, as is seen in comparing the first and second outbreaks. The first epidemic had lower case–fatality ratios than the second (13·4% and 60% respectively), and the onset of clinical illness was also generally less fulminant. In the first outbreak, the cap-liners were contaminated at the time of manufacture, but most fluids probably remained free of contamination until the caps were removed in preparation for administration. Thus, in most instances, probably few microorganisms were infused during the first several hours of intravenous therapy. In contrast, contaminants were apparently introduced directly into fluid at the time of manufacture in the second outbreak, and the contaminants had time to proliferate before infusion was started. Additionally, the underlying illness of the patient affects clinical outcome; in the first outbreak, patients with an ultimately fatal illness had a 44·2% fatality rate attributed to the bacteraemia while patients with non-fatal underlying illnesses had a 7·4% rate[1].

I have incomplete follow-up information on patients who survived these episodes of septicaemia, but I am not aware of frequent late or metastatic infections in these patients. While we have seen metastatic infections complicating nosocomial bacteraemia with both Gram-positive and Gram-negative microorganisms, I know of no cases of endocarditis or osteomyelitis as complications of these outbreaks in the United States.

To summarize the clinical characteristics associated with infusion of intrinsically contaminated intravenous fluid, several points must be re-emphasized (Table 8.2). Most important, there are no clinical clues that

TABLE 8.2   **Clinical characteristics of infusion bacteraemia**

1. Typical Gram-negative septicaemia
2. Patients without obvious predisposition
3. Clinical outcome influenced by management of contaminated fluid

are *diagnostic* of intrinsic contamination. Most patients have illnesses quite compatible with bacterial septicaemia arising from any source. And although the characteristics listed in Table 8.2 are suggestive of infusion-related bacteraemia, they occur with intrinsically contaminated infusions as well as extrinsically contaminated infusion fluid, drip-set or catheter site sepsis. Thus, if intrinsic contamination is to be recognized promptly and dealt with appropriately, other clues are needed. In the United States, we believe that the epidemiological syndrome of intrinsic contamination provides such clues.

8.2.2 Epidemiology

Each episode of infusion contamination in the United States was recognized because of a significant increase in the incidence of primary bacteraemia‡ in an affected hospital. Figure 8.1 shows the occurrence of pseudomonas

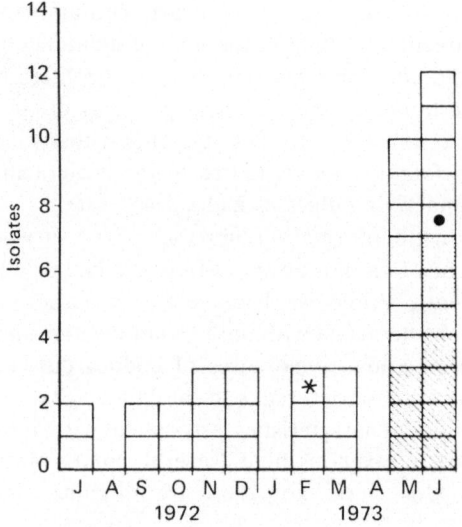

*Only the first isolate from any one patient is tabulated

▢ *Pseudomonas* species isolate sensitive only
to chloramphenicol and tetracycline

▢ *Pseudomonas* species isolate with growth characteristics
that did not permit sensitivity determinations

▢ *Pseudomonas aeruginosa* isolate

✳ *Pseudomonas* species, no antibiogram performed

● *Pseudomonas* species sensitive only to carbenicillin,
gentamicin, chloramphenicol, and tetracycline

Figure 8.1 *Pseudomonas* spp. blood isolates, University Hospital, by month of isolation

‡ 'Primary bacteraemia' is defined as bacteraemia thought to be related to intravenous therapy or bacteraemia not attributable to recognized infection at another site within the patient

bacteraemia in the university hospital that first recognized the third epidemic. Before May 1973, non-aeruginosa pseudomonas blood isolates were found only rarely. In May and June there was a striking increase in such isolates, and this increase prompted an epidemiological investigation that incriminated intrinsically contaminated albumin infusions. Similar observations had occurred in each of the other outbreaks and led to the solution of the problem.

Surveillance in a single hospital, however, may not be sufficiently sensitive to recognize low-frequency contamination, such as where only one out of every 1000 units is contaminated, or where a product is used only infrequently. In such circumstances, discovery of an occasional case of disease might not be sufficient to cause alarm. The lack of sensitivity of clinical surveillance can be minimized by combining data from many institutions.

Figure 8.2 shows the incidence of *Enterobacter* bacteraemia in 49 hospitals in the United States that report regularly as part of the National Nosocomial Infections Study (NNIS). This study has since 1970 collected nosocomial infection surveillance data from voluntarily participating hospitals[6]. As early as July 1970, the incidence of *Enterobacter* bacteraemia rose above levels previously seen and this elevated incidence persisted, and even increased, until contaminated fluids were withdrawn from use in March 1971. When the 49 hospitals were grouped according to their sources of intravenous fluid during the epidemic period, the increase in *Enterobacter* bacteraemia cases was entirely accounted for by hospitals

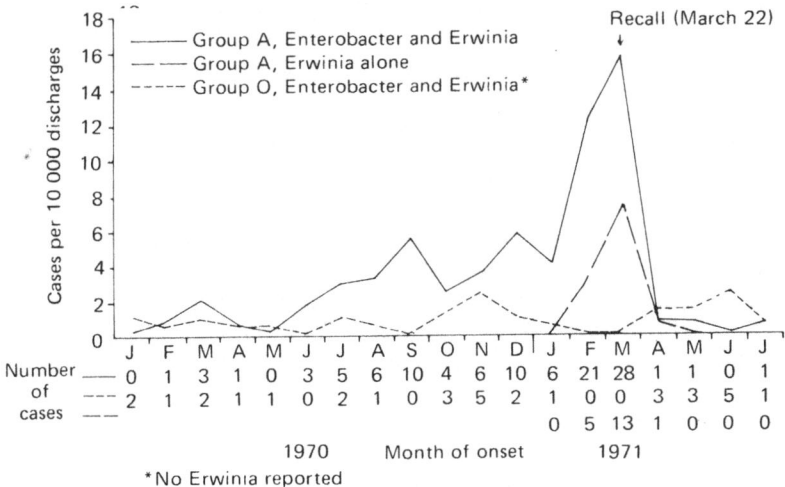

Figure 8.2 Incidence of primary *Enterobacter* and *Erwinia* bacteraemia in all regularly reporting NNIS hospitals

using fluids from the implicated manufacturer[7]. Several of the hospitals contributing to the excess number of reported cases of bacteraemia had only sporadic cases early in the epidemic, but when their data are combined with data from other hospitals, the epidemic is clearly apparent.

Second, the involved pathogens have not caused epidemic disease at other clinical sites such as urinary or respiratory tracts. The absence of epidemic disease at these other sites suggests that the bacteraemia is truly primary and not related to a more generalized infection problem in the hospital.

Third, each recognized outbreak has involved few microbial species. Having an epidemic with only a single strain does not exclude extrinsic contamination of intravenous fluids, but it does make intrinsic contamination more likely, since extrinsic contamination often occurs with a variety of different strains.

Fourth, recognized outbreaks have thus far involved relatively unusual blood isolates such as *E. cloacae*, *E. agglomerans*, *C. freundii*, and *P. cepacia*. This, in part, reflects the relatively narrow spectrum of micro-organisms that can thrive in infusion fluids[8,9], but it may also reflect the greater difficulty of detecting low-frequency contamination with more common pathogens. *Klebsiella* spp., for example, also proliferate in dextrose-containing fluid[8], but they have not yet been shown to cause an outbreak of disease due to intrinsic contamination in the United States.

Fifth, in several of the outbreaks, the isolates have had unusually sensitive antimicrobial susceptibility patterns. Gram-negative pathogens isolated from nosocomial infections typically are resistant *in vitro* to a variety of antimicrobial agents perhaps as a result of selective pressures imposed by the use of antibiotics in the hospital. It is unusual to find a very sensitive strain causing epidemic disease; such a finding suggests a possible non-hospital reservoir for the epidemic strain. In these epidemics, those reservoirs were the manufacturing plants.

These five clues suggest intrinsic contamination of an infusion product, but further supportive evidence requires an epidemiological investigation. In such an investigation, one expects to find a highly significant association between disease among patients in a hospital and exposure to a specific infusion product. Finally, intrinsic contamination is strongly suggested if a similar epidemic pattern can be documented in more than one hospital using the same fluids but cannot be documented in hospitals using other products.

The experience in Great Britain with one outbreak[10] suggested that contaminated fluids are turbid to careful inspection. In the three out-breaks that we investigated, neither fluids contaminated at manufacture nor fluids artificially inoculated with epidemic strains in our laboratory have shown turbidity. Thus, turbidity if present is evidence of contamination, but we cannot rely upon the simple technique of visual inspection of fluid bottles to recognize intrinsic contamination.

In an effort to discover intrinsic contamination before patients are exposed to products, some hospitals have embarked on extensive sterility sampling of commercially-acquired products. However, if appropriate quality control procedures are followed by the manufacturers of these products, such expensive procedures are not necessary unless a clinical outbreak is suspected. The seven features discussed below (Table 8.3) have been characteristic of outbreaks thus far recognized and offer guidance in the evaluation of future potential epidemics, but it would be shortsighted to rely upon efficient recognition of patient disease as the prime safeguard against intrinsic contamination of parenteral fluids. Instead, we should seek ways to prevent contamination in the first place. And for this, we must look to the manufacturers of these products.

TABLE 8.3   Epidemiological characteristics of bacteraemia caused by intrinsic contamination of infusion products

1. Increased incidence of PRIMARY bacteraemia
2. No alteration in disease incidence at other sites
3. Single—or only a few—species of microorganism responsible
4. Unusual pathogen often responsible
5. Unusual sensitivity pattern
6. Significant association with infusion therapy
7. Similar episodes in other hospitals

8.3 MANUFACTURERS' RESPONSIBILITIES

The manufacturer of a therapeutic agent bears the ultimate responsibility for producing a sterile product. Although the episodes of recognized intrinsic contamination have been few, the epidemics that have occurred suggest that quality control over the manufacture of infusion products has, in the past, been less than perfect.

Two basic approaches have been used by the pharmaceutical industry to prevent release of contaminated products. The first, which we might call 'process control', focuses upon management of the production process in order to prevent contamination. For example, the sterilization process is carefully monitored with biological indicators within each autoclave load, and the temperature and pressure within the autoclave are further monitored electronically. Based upon carefully developed theoretical considerations, such processes have been claimed to be sufficient to assure that sterilization fails no more often than in one unit out of every 10 million produced. Improvements in such process controls have been the major interest of both industry and the US Food and Drug Administration (FDA).

The second approach, a more traditional safeguard, is end-product sterility testing. Here, a proportion of the finished product is sampled and cultured microbiologically. If the sample of finished units is sterile on culture, and the sample selected from the product at the termination of the manufacturing process is sterile, there is added assurance that the manufacturing process, including process controls, has been effective. A positive culture, on the other hand, may reflect either intrinsic contamination—i.e., a failure of process controls—or adventitial contamination introduced at the time of sampling—i.e., a false-positive test result. Knowing the identity of the organisms as well as their concentration in the fluid will help you judge the likelihood of having a false-positive result and evaluate the potential public health seriousness of the observation.

Many manufacturers in the United States routinely perform sterility testing of finished products, but they are not required to do so by law or regulation at the present time. Since the presence or absence of microbial adulteration is legally decided on the basis of United States Pharmacopeia (USP) test procedures, and thus it is prudent for manufacturers to employ USP sterility tests. However some have claimed that sterility testing is inefficient and that USP sterility tests should be de-emphasized or even discarded.

The opposition to sterility testing is based on a statistical argument. Figure 8.3 shows that the probability of detecting contamination is a function of the sample size. Since one must destroy a bottle of intravenous fluid in order to culture it with currently available techniques, it is most important to take no more samples for testing than absolutely necessary. But the figure shows that for a typical batch of products, low level contamination is unlikely to be detected short of almost destructive sampling of the entire production batch. For example, if 1% of a production batch is contaminated, a 1% sampling of the batch gives a mere 5% chance of obtaining a positive culture; with a 5% sample, the odds are improved, but one would still detect contamination in fewer than half the tests. To be assured of a positive test at the 95% confidence level, one would have to sample approximately half the finished products. Clearly, this is economically impractical unless we are to inflate the price of infusion products beyond reason.

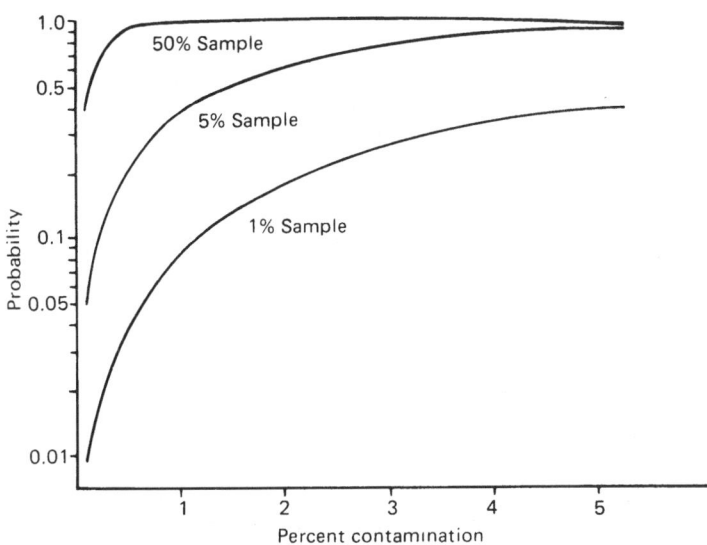

Figure 8.3 Probabilities of detecting contamination as functions of percentage contamination and proportion of products sampled

The statistical basis for this argument rests upon several faulty assumptions, however. First, the argument assumes that process controls are as efficient as an economically feasible sampling scheme in preventing distribution of a contaminated product. However, the history of outbreaks both in the United States and Great Britain shows that recognized epidemics have not resulted from failures in sterilization, but because of contamination introduced after the last step of the sterilization process was completed. Therefore, even if the sterilization process were 100% reliable, none of the US epidemics would have been prevented. Furthermore, the argument assumes that we can design safe production lines. Again, experience suggests otherwise. For in two of the US outbreaks, contamination was seemingly facilitated by relatively minor changes in the production process that did not seem, *a priori*, to increase the risk of contamination. Thus, unless we completely understand all production factors affecting product sterility, it does not seem prudent to rely on process controls alone.

Finally, and most importantly, the argument against product sampling is based upon assessments of its value for finding contamination in a single contaminated batch. It ignores the fact that contamination in the United

TABLE 8.4 Probabilities of detecting contamination at various levels by sampling five units per 1000 produced

Units made (thousands)	Autoclave loads	contamination rate					
		1/10 000		1/1000		6/1000	
		No. of contaminated units produced	Probability one or more detected	No. of contaminated units produced	Probability one or more detected	No. of contaminated units produced	Probability one or more detected
33·4	3·3	3	0·02	33	0·15	200	0·63
100	10	10	0·05	100	0·39	600	0·95
200	20	20	0·10	200	0·63		
300	30	30	0·14	300	0·78		
400	40	40	0·18	400	0·86		
500	50	50	0·22	500	0·92		
600	60	60	0·26	600	0·95		
750	75	75	0·31				
1000	100	100	0·39				
2000	200	200	0·63				
4000	400	400	0·86				
6000	600	600	0·95				

States has typically occurred at very low rates and affected numerous batches produced over a prolonged period of time. The fact that multiple production batches may be contaminated has a major impact on the true statistical value of sampling, and the probability calculations in Figure 8.3 are not appropriate for such settings.

To illustrate this, let us consider a hypothetical example. Assume that a manufacturer has one autoclave that will sterilize 10 000 bottles in a batch. Further assume that because of a continuing problem in the autoclave, one bottle of each 10 000 unit lot is always contaminated. Let us then sample an economically feasible portion of the load; 5 units of each 1000 or a total of 50 units randomly selected from each batch. The first four left-hand columns of Table 8.4 show what we can expect as we continue to sample batches. Early on, one stands a miniscule chance of detecting contamination; even after three loads have been sampled, there is but a 2% chance of having detected contamination. As production continues, however, the *cumulative* probability of obtaining at least one positive culture from our random sampling increases so that by the time 200 contaminated units have been produced, there is a 63% chance of obtaining a positive culture; and by the time a mere 600 contaminated units have been produced, there is a greater than 95% chance of detecting the contamination. Thus, the results of end-product sampling will reflect continuing low levels of contamination.

The next two columns in the table show what we can expect if contamination occurs more frequently. Here, 10 units per batch of 10 000 are contaminated; at the same sampling rate—five bottles per 1000 produced—we more quickly reach the 95% confidence level that contamination will have been detected. But note that, as with the previous level of contamination, it is highly (95%) probable that detection will have occurred by the time 600 contaminated units have been produced. As further illustrated by the final columns, the probability of detecting contamination is linked with the total number of contaminated units that are produced, and this relationship is not influenced by the ongoing rate of product contamination although it is influenced by the sampling fraction.

It is my purpose here not to propose a specific sampling scheme but rather to stress two important points. First, an economically feasible sample taken for culture is not likely to document contamination if the contamination affects only a small number of units in a single batch; but if numerous batches are affected, as has been the general rule, the probabilities of detecting contamination accumulate over time and can virtually assure detection using practically feasible sampling fractions before large numbers of contaminated products have been distributed for use. Second, this illustration directs us to our real concern; the numbers of contaminated units actually distributed for use. It is just as dangerous to allow distribution of 1000 batches each containing one contaminated unit as it is to allow distribution of a single batch containing 1000 tainted bottles. Equal numbers of patients are placed at risk of disease or death. Any system used to prevent product contamination should be equally effective in detecting and preventing either of these situations.

In the example that I used, a total production of 600 contaminated units could be detected with 95% confidence. If one were willing to pay the cost of taking larger sampling fractions, one could reasonably assure detection of fewer contaminated units. Thus, the decision about the number of samples to take becomes a question of 'cost-benefit' that can be answered by balancing the costs of disease against the costs of sampling. Lest we recoil at the thought of placing human life and death in such economic terms, let me stress that manufacturers can *guarantee* sterility of every unit only if they culture, and thereby destroy, every unit. So the cost-benefit question cannot be avoided; rather, it must be approached in the most rational manner available.

Finally, the hypothetical sampling system that I have described should not be viewed as a specific proposal since it is relatively unsophisticated. For example, it does not differentiate between a problem in a single batch and ongoing production defect when a single positive culture is obtained. But such an objective may be approached by applying sequential sampling concepts to develop a procedure that incorporates the past history of quality control results in deciding whether unacceptable rates of intrinsic contamination are likely to be present.

8.4 CONCLUSIONS

The administration of intravenous infusion fluids is now a remarkably safe therapeutic practice. There are, however, hazards. Of infectious hazards, I submit that extrinsic contamination of infusion systems (including both the cannula and the drip-set) is a major problem to be dealt with. However, the spectre of intrinsic contamination continues to haunt our use of these systems. Intrinsic contamination probably continuously occurs at rates sufficiently low to produce no recognizable epidemiological problem, and at rates that would only very rarely result in rejection of a particular autoclave load by current sterility testing procedures. When it has occurred at higher rates, a vast population of hospitalized patients has sometimes been placed in jeopardy.

As long as epidemic nosocomial infections remain a threat, we must maintain vigilant surveillance for patient disease. The benefits of surveillance have been demonstrated by the recognition of epidemics in the United States and Great Britain. However, surveillance merely recognizes disease after it has occurred. It does not automatically identify the source of disease and, as with bacteraemia resulting from intrinsic contamination of infusion products, the source is occasionally difficult to document. Furthermore, surveillance is often incomplete and may only reveal a fragment of true cases, thus delaying the recognition of a problem or totally missing a very low frequency event.

As a result, our principal goal must be to institute the most sensitive controls possible over the manufacturing processes. Our currently available technological resources do not allow us to prevent intrinsic contamination. We can, however, minimize the risk of its occurrence. This will require not only improvements in the actual production of components of infusion systems, it will also require a sensitive assessment of the microbiological properties of those components. While substantial progress continues to be made in improving production processes, I am concerned about the tendency to discount the importance of end-product sterility testing. I am convinced that a sequential sampling system to monitor the production process, as alluded to above, is not only economically practical but is also scientifically practical. There may also be other schemes equally or better suited to these tasks. Until rational end-product sterility testing is uniformly adopted by manufacturers of sterile medical products, we will be dependent on surveillance of patients to detect contamination. This seems to me most inappropriate; for, despite the acknowledged costs of an effective sterility testing programme, test tubes are still less precious than people.

Acknowledgements

Drs Dennis G. Maki, Frank S. Rhame, Donald A. Goldmann, James H. Tenney, and Allen C. Steere, Jr participated in the epidemiological investigations reported. Dr John V. Bennett supervised the work reported herein and was of great assistance in the preparation of this manuscript.

References

1. Maki, D. G., Rhame, F. S., Mackel, D. C. and Bennett, J. V. (1976). Nationwide epidemic of septicemia caused by contaminated intravenous products. I. Epidemiologic and clinical features. *Am. J. Med.*, **60**, 471

2. Center for Disease Control. (1973). Septicemias associated with contaminated intravenous fluids—Wisconsin, Ohio. *Morbid. Mortal. Weekly Rep.*, **22**, 99
3. Center for Disease Control. (1973). Follow-up on septicemias associated with contaminated intravenous fluids—United States. *Morbid. Mortal. Weekly Rep.*, **22**, 115
4. Center for Disease Control. (1973). Nosocomial *Pseudomonas* spp. bacteremias—Maryland. *Morbid. Mortal. Weekly Rep.*, **22**, 265
5. Bennett, J. V. (1975). Presentation recorded in minutes of the Proceedings of the Panel on End-Product Sterility Testing, USP, November 25
6. Bennett, J. V., Scheckler, W. E., Maki, D. G. and Brachman, P. S. (1971). Current national patterns—United States. In P. S. Brachman and T. C. Eickhoff (eds). *Proceedings of the International Conference on Nosocomial Infections*, pp. 42–49. (Chicago: American Hospital Association)
7. Center for Disease Control. (1972). Nationwide epidemic of septicemia associated with intravenous fluid therapy: an analysis based on the CDC National Nosocomial Infections Study. *National Nosocomial Infections Study, Report* (Issued October 1972), p. 23
8. Maki, D. G. and Martin, W. T. (1975). Nationwide epidemic of septicemia caused by contaminated infusion products. IV. Growth of microbial pathogens in fluids for intravenous infusion. *J. Infect. Dis.*, **131**, 267
9. Goldmann, D. A., Martin, W. T. and Worthington, J. W. (1973). Growth of bacteria and fungi in total parenteral nutrition solutions. *Am. J. Surg.*, **126**, 314
10. Meers, P. D., Calder, M. W., Mazhar, M. M. and Lawrie, G. M. (1973). Intravenous infusion of contaminated dextrose solution. The Devonport incident. *Lancet*, **ii**, 1189

DISCUSSION

Clinical problems and epidemiology
Panel: P. F. D'Arcy (in the chair)
R. E. Dixon, A. M. Geddes,
B. S. Jenkins and D. G. Maki

1 ADDITIVES

Dr T. J. BRADLEY (Birmingham): Many hospital pharmacies have good sterile working areas where additions of drugs to solutions for intravenous injection can be made. However, there are many hospitals that do not have such facilities, yet the pharmacist is still capable of monitoring this particular exercise.

Would Dr Geddes comment on pharmacists in such hospitals coming on to the wards and carrying out drug additions to intravenous fluids and preparing solutions ready for injection in a ward?

I believe that there are certain legal implications, but it would be very valuable for pharmacists to have an opinion.

Dr GEDDES (Birmingham): The ward pharmacy system is undoubtedly a major advance in hospital pharmacy services. Our own ward pharmacists do advise on additives, and we encourage them to educate the nursing staff and the junior medical staff. As to the ward pharmacist making the additions, at present the ward pharmacist usually has a large number of wards to cover, and can visit the wards once, or at the most twice, in a day. Many of the additives are best added with as short a period as possible between addition and administration to the patient.

The problem is that at the moment hospital pharmacy services are generally 9 am to 5 pm services, and that is really the crux of the matter. The ideal would be a 24-hour 7-days-a-week service, and then it might be practical to have it all done in the pharmacy.

One of the problems is that many, if not the majority, of acute admissions to hospital come in during the late afternoon. The busiest time is often between 4 and 8 pm, and that is the time when the service is often not available.

Dr MAKI (Madison, Wisconsin): In the United States there has been a considerable thrust towards the centralization of pharmacy admixture programmes even to the point where the pharmacist is on the ward frequently to prepare admixtures. In most programmes however, admixtures are prepared in a central part of the hospital, particularly in laminar flow hood facilities and under optimal conditions of asepsis; this is particularly true of programmes compounding solutions for total parenteral nutrition.

There are major advantages in having a pharmacist prepare all intravenous admixtures. It is unfair to ask the nurse to be a person for all seasons, specifically also to be an expert in clinical pharmacy. The pharmacist prepares most drugs. Intravenous fluids should be thought of as drugs, and in my opinion should be compounded by a pharmacist whenever possible.

The single theoretical concern with the central pharmacy admixture service is that there is a potential for common source outbreaks* if there is a breakdown in aseptic technique in the pharmacy. However, the advantages to be gained, particularly in the non-microbiological sphere— e.g., minimizing drug errors and minimizing drug interactions—I believe outweigh this hazard. The pharmacist can play an extremely valuable role in intercepting an order that could potentially prove hazardous to the patient.

In the area of infection control, as I mentioned previously, there may be less contamination by Gram-negative bacilli with pharmacy-prepared solutions. Reservoirs of Gram-negative bacilli are rife all over the ward, but theoretically they are not in the pharmacy. These organisms are the ones which cause problems in solutions due to their ability to proliferate in parenteral fluids.†

The National Coordinating Committee on Large Volume Parenterals in the United States, sponsored by the Food and Drug Administration and the USP, recently went formally on record recommending that all admixtures that are prepared electively in hospitals, with the exception of emergencies, be prepared by a central pharmacy admixture service in a centrally designated area of the hospital‡. This will probably be incorporated into the recommendations of the USA Joint Commission on Accreditation of Hospitals. It would not surprise me to see the percentage of US hospitals with central pharmacy admixture services jump from the current 25–30% to near 100% within the next five to ten years.

Dr BRADLEY: There are recommendations within the UK that where the pharmacist is professionally involved, he should carry out the drug additions and admixtures in a sterile working area. Nevertheless in the ward he still has the same knowledge and the same skills, although the conditions are different.

Many drug additions for intravenous administration take place on the wards and are made by unskilled junior hospital doctors or nursing staff. The pharmacist has the necessary skills. Why should these be confined to the hospital pharmacy?

Dr MAKI: I am not suggesting that he should be confined. In my own hospital the pharmacists are on the wards and often go to the bedside

* See Chapter 7, reference 37a
† See Chapter 2, reference 15
‡ See Chapter 7, reference 111

and administer intravenous medication. The ward is the appropriate place for many of their activities.

Professor D'ARCY (Belfast): But it has to be a 24-hour service, and it has to cover the weekend, and not stop at 5 o'clock on a Friday.

Dr BRADLEY: That would be a goal to work towards.

Professor D'ARCY: No it is not! Nursing staff cannot be told to cover from 5 o'clock on Friday afternoon until 9 o'clock on Monday morning whilst the pharmacist does it during the week. That is absolutely impossible.

I am speaking also in my capacity as Chairman of a Nursing School, which has objected most strongly to the attitude of: 'Oh, yes; you'll do it when it is convenient to you, and we'll have to do it when you're away'. That is not the way to do it. Either it is a 24-hour service, or it is not at all.

In the survey that we did in Ulster (D'Arcy, P. F. and Thompson, K. M. (1974). *Pharm. J.*, **213**, 178), we showed that drug additions were made in equal numbers from 9 am to 5 pm as from 5 pm to 9 am, and the number from 5 pm to midnight was much the same as from midnight to 5 am. It was almost constant throughout the 24 hours.

Mr N. GEE (Burnley): Over the past three years we have proved that it can be done on a 24-hour basis, including weekends, with a normal pharmacy staff. We tend to do one weekend a month, which we do not find too taxing, and we find that the service has been welcomed by both medical and nursing staff. We have been able to eliminate the incompatibilities that were there when we began, and to standardize throughout the whole system.

2 INTRAVENOUS THERAPY TEAM

Dr E. MITCHELL (London): We should like to hear more about the team that Dr Maki described, the number of people, their qualifications, the scope and numbers of patients, the size of a team for a thousand-bed hospital, and so on.

Dr MAKI: The concept of the intravenous therapy team is based on the proven success of the team approach to management of infusions for total parenteral nutrition. As with any therapy that is newly introduced, total parenteral nutrition was probably grossly over-used, and as such abused in its early years. It was introduced in about 1969, or 1970, and in the early years of total parenteral nutrition in the US the experience with infection was abysmal. There were rates of related septicaemia in hospitals that were as high as 25–30%. It is difficult to countenance a therapeutic modality for patients with reversible diseases what has a 25–30% incidence of septicaemia, particularly with *Candida*, which is often fatal.

Looking at the situation critically, it was apparent that the problem was that the unique susceptibility of the patients to infection from these catheters was not perceived. (As discussed, sepsis in TPN is really the extreme of all catheter-related infection.) It was realized that medical personnel were drawing blood through the lines, giving blood products and all kinds of medication through them, and even using them to take central venous pressure measurements. The catheter sites were specifically not getting any special care.

When the necessity for the uncompromising standard of care that is required to take care of TPN catheters became obvious, the infection rate dropped precipitously, and this has now been well documented in a number of hospitals in the US. Many large US institutions employ a team approach to TPN. No one is allowed to touch the catheter, other than the very limited number of people with responsibility for it, i.e., team members. They check the site at least every other day, sometimes daily. Most importantly, they look at the patient every day. At the onset of any unexplained fever they obtain blood cultures and may well elect to remove the catheter. With this approach, TPN can be delivered with a rate of complicating infection of 1 or 2% and in some institutions, as low as 0% per 100 infusions.

This team approach was obviously successful in TPN, and has now given great impetus in the US to the concept of intravenous therapy teams for the management of all parenteral infusions in the hospital. As a consequence many institutions in the US have established teams, generally consisting of registered nurses or licensed practical nurses. In some institutions they may include medical technologists. These individuals are trained to insert peripheral venous cannulae. They use needles wherever possible, or else small plastic catheters. They do not generally insert central venous pressure lines, or jugular or subclavian catheters. In some institutions they may insert radial artery catheters, but this is uncommon. They are trained to insert cannulae under the most uniform standards of asepsis possible. They usually have their own materials that they carry around with them.

The most valuable service they provide in my opinion is not just the uniform standard of asepsis that can be brought to insertion of a catheter, but the follow-up surveillance. The greatest hazard of cannula-related infection, or any infusion-related infection, is when the infusion is 'forgotten'—when the potential iatrogenic hazards are not appreciated and the catheter stays in for a prolonged period of time.

A typical situation is of a patient who comes out of an intensive care unit. He was initially critically ill, and expected to die. Three days later he has stabilized, is looking better and is transferred to the ward. No one on the ward notices that the subclavian catheter that was used for central venous pressure measurements has already been in for 72 hours. It's 'convenient' to leave it in because the patient needs further parenteral antibiotics for his pneumococcal meningitis. Several days later the patient develops a catheter-related staphylococcal septicaemia.

A team permits uncompromising surveillance of *every* intravenous infusion in the hospital. Every patient can be seen every day. It is not necessary to examine the infusion site every day, but the team can check for complaints of pain, for a red streak rising up the arm, for unexplained fever. If the answer to any of those questions is yes, or if the catheter has been in for more than 2–3 days, they will take it out and in a suspect situation, also culture the catheter.

The advantages of a team are six-fold:

1. Promote the use of steel needles in preference to catheters because people are available to replace cannulae more frequently.

2. Assure that plastic catheters are removed reliably within 48–72 hours.

3. Identify infusion-related septicaemia more rapidly; if the patient has unexplained fever, a team member is available to take out the suspect catheter and culture it and obtain blood cultures.

4. Recognize potential epidemic problems, that can be very insidious, more rapidly and reliably. The team looks in on all patients receiving intravenous therapy, and should immediately recognize a cluster of two or more infusion-related septicaemias that may auger an outbreak.

5. An intravenous therapy team can permit the smallest hospital to adopt a scholarly approach to intravenous therapy. They can prospectively evaluate any new infection control measure, such as a new cannula, a new topical antibiotic or a new anaesthetic, in a controlled fashion. The fifty-bed hospital with a one- or two-person team can do it.

6. Facilitate education of personnel in safe techniques of infusion therapy.

The intravenous therapy team is probably most important in a large hospital, with its very large and tremendously heterogeneous population of individuals participating in intravenous therapy.

I emphasize that I am not suggesting that the intravenous therapy team is the only answer, or the ultimate answer to reliable asepsis in infusion therapy. But in real life, in a large hospital, it is very hard to provide a uniform standard of care for infusion therapy. This has been my experience in three institutions. I have seen many catheter-related septicaemias. In most institutions with intravenous therapy teams extraordinarily low rates of catheter-related infection are generally found, despite the fact that team members are specifically looking for iatrogenic infection.

Dr MITCHELL: How many nurses, and reporting to whom?

Dr MAKI: In my own hospital we hope to implement a team in July 1976. We have a 600-bed hospital, and to start with we shall try to cover from 80–85% of the adult beds in the hospital. We have done some time-utilization studies, and we expect to cover 85% of the hospital, seven days a week, for 18 hours a day, with a team of four persons. There will be 6 hours each night when the team will not cover the hospital, but we have found that less than 5% of all cannulae are started in that 6-hour period. The team members will report to the Assistant Director of the Pharmacy and to me. We will be the co-directors of the team.

Dr GEDDES: The questions asked by both Dr Bradley and Dr Mitchell have medico-legal undertones. There is some concern that the pharmacist adding drugs to bottles in the ward may not have medico-legal backing should a mistake occur. It goes back to the training of hospital pharmacists. I personally have little doubt that hospital pharmacists should receive a different training from retail pharmacists. If they were properly trained for the job, there would be no medico-legal implications.

In my own hospital we have just won the battle to allow trained nurses in intensive care units and in certain other specialized units to undertake venepuncture to remove blood. The next stage is likely to be an approach to Dr Maki's concept. I would agree that a well-trained sister is probably much better at putting up a drip than a newly-qualified houseman.

Dr BRADLEY: There are medical procedures set up and approved, and that is a very good defence for a doctor in the event of an incident. Similar procedures have been set up for nurses. However, the pharmacist carrying out work on the ward is in a situation which is new, and set procedures have perhaps not been agreed.

My concern is that in those hospitals which do not have sterile working facilities, the pharmacist's expertise is not being utilized. Obviously we should aim for a 24-hour service, and for good conditions, but the process has to start somewhere. The skills that the pharmacist has should be put to use in training nurses or monitoring systems. With the advice and the backing of a good ward pharmacy scheme, such as the scheme operating in East Birmingham that Dr Geddes described, this sounds an ideal place to start.

Professor D'ARCY: It seems to end with, and to start with, education. The training of the pharmacist needs to be changed to do precisely the job that we are discussing. To be critical of the academic pharmacy course, it does not currently include that type of training.

Mr J. A. WANDLESS (London): The role of the Drugs and the Therapeutics Committees in American hospitals is to look after the interests of the patient in respect of drugs in use in the hospitals. Is the team described by Dr Maki responsible to the Drug and Therapeutics Committee in his own hospital?

Secondly, Dr Maki mentioned accreditation, and expressed the hope that the team he described will become part of the accreditation system in the hospitals. Did I understand that correctly?

Dr MAKI: No. It seems logical that a team is the most reliable approach for safe intravenous therapy, but I should not be so presumptuous as to state that this team should be the standard for accreditation. Intravenous therapy teams have not yet been scientifically proven by controlled trial as the best approach, and there is obviously also the cost-benefit aspect.

Coming back to the first question, the intravenous therapy team would answer to the Pharmacy and Therapeutics Committee and the Infection Control Committee.

3   DRIP-SITE INFECTION

Mr F. DURNING (Derby): Sources of contamination with intravenous drips have been mentioned. What about the cover that is put on to retain the catheter? Sometimes sterile gauze is used, and sometimes Elastoplast.

Dr MAKI: If I am asked to recommend what I should use on top of the catheter, I can say what I personally use, but I know of no good studies on the optimal type of cover.

I use a 4×4 inch sterile gauze pad, double strength. I first apply an antimicrobial ointment to the site, then fold in the gauze underneath the external portion of the catheter to lift it away from the skin, and then tape it down. I am easily able to remove the dressing every other day to look at the site and to reapply ointment if it is necessary to leave the catheter in place for longer than 48 hours.

Mr G. SYKES (London): What ointment is used?

Dr MAKI: In total parenteral nutrition we have been using iodophor ointment. With conventional infusion therapy we have been using a combination antibiotic ointment containing polymyxin, neomycin and bacitracin.

Mrs H. M. DULSON (Crawley): Dr Geddes was rather critical of nurses, and he mentioned dirty scissors to open intravenous containers. There are two other areas of malpractice on which I should like to comment.

First, often the vein is cleaned in the accepted manner, and then a rather dubious index finger is used to find the vein. Secondly there is the use of the serum, or other needle, to maintain an airway in plastic intravenous infusion containers.

Dr GEDDES: I hope that I was no more critical of nurses than I was of my medical colleagues. I shared the criticism equally, or attempted to do so.

I entirely agree that doctors putting up drips frequently do not even wash their hands. They may claim that they are not touching the site of insertion of the needle, but they often fiddle about to find the vein, and anyone who has watched the insertion of needles and cannulae will admit that it can be a very difficult procedure; it may take a long time and be fraught with increasing frustration. The risk of contamination prospects probably increases linearly with the frustration! I have seen the needle dropped on to the floor, or on the bedclothes, and then inserted.

In answer to the question about sticking a needle into the top of a container, I would say that it is quite unnecessary, although it may have been needed with earlier and more rigid packs. There are people who feel that sticking a needle into the top will cause the drip to run more quickly. It is a dangerous practice because it sucks in unsterile air. We have certainly managed to stop it in our hospital, by education and discipline.

Could I correct a possible misunderstanding regarding something to which Dr Jenkins referred. I am not against central venous pressure monitoring in an intensive care unit under the eye of someone who understands it, but I am against central venous pressure monitoring carried out by the houseman in the corner of the general ward.

Dr G. AYLIFFE (Birmingham): We use a different method to Dr Maki for detecting drip-site infection but we have often isolated a pathogen from the broth alone, such as a klebsiella, and yet found nothing in the original plate, so quantitative cultures are important.

Dr MAKI: What does it mean when the klebsiella is positive in the broth, and not in the plate?

Dr AYLIFFE: It probably means very little, and we tend to ignore it. There is still a problem of interpretation, but it does help quite considerably.

We have also been looking at the changing of drip sets, and catheters. Perhaps 30% of catheters are not changed after two days, and the drip set figures seem to be about the same, which would suggest that they are left in all the time. It will probably be extremely expensive to change drip sets after one day. Can it be validated in terms of infection?

Dr MAKI: I tried to make the point that there is no good answer on the optimal period for change. Deriving an interval which is rational economically and will also be effective in terms of protecting the patient from contamination is exceedingly difficult, because sepsis due to contamination of fluid is probably a low-frequency event. A 48-hour change may turn out not to be optimal, but is at present reasonable since we do not have better information. We changed giving-sets every 24 hours at the height of the 1970–71 US Abbott epidemic*, because we had a major problem, and this interval was effective in diminishing epidemic septicaemias. Many US hospitals, including my own, now utilize 48 hours as the interval, and it may turn out that an even longer interval such as 72 hours is sufficient because contamination with dangerous pathogens, i.e. with growth potential, is fortunately comparatively infrequent.

Mr J. A. MYERS (Edinburgh): Dr Maki referred to plastic cannulae several times, but there are a number of different plastics, some quite inert. He did not specify which plastic cannulae. They come in different shapes, some easier to insert, and some more difficult to insert.

We also heard that needles might be the panacea. Do needles become coated with a fibrin coat after a day or so?

Dr MAKI: No one knows the answer to that. There have been a number of studies of the fibrin sleeve, with plastic catheters, primarily angiographic studies. They do an angiogram with the catheter in the vein, or in the artery and have conclusive findings, but I know of no comparable angiographic study done with needles. I have no idea whether a clot forms,

* See Chapter 7, reference 4

or if so, with what frequency. However, needles appear to be substantially safer than plastic catheters.

I know of no data pertaining to differences in infection rates among different types of plastic. I do not think that anyone knows whether the material makes a difference. Data exist on phlebitis, in terms of the effect of catheter material, but here they are in conflict. There are now available in the US smaller plastic catheters, one inch or so long, as compared to the larger bore three to twelve inch catheters which were employed in most published studies of catheter-related infection. These smaller catheters may be substantially safer. I have seen only a couple of cases of septicaemia with them, (and these small catheters are the main plastic catheters used in our hospitals) whereas I have seen comparatively many more cases of septicaemia with the old longer plastic catheters.

Mr G. HUGHES (Canterbury): Has Dr Maki investigated the cannula in haemodialysis patients, and the relative incidence of infection there?

Secondly, have two-way taps any place in infusion equipment?

Dr MAKI: I ran out of time to discuss taps. It would seem logical that they would present a substantial hazard. They are frequently covered by dried intravenous fluid, and they are frequently grossly soiled by dried blood. I know of one investigator who has cultured the inner surface and found occasional Gram-negative bacilli*, but she did no cultures of fluid, and provided no clinical correlations in terms of disease, so I would not know what that contamination means. People talk about taps, and allude to them in the literature, but I know of no hard data that quantifies their risk. It is the same with all the factors in the infusion. It makes sense to avoid taps. They are another potential source of trouble and they should not be incorporated in the system unless there is a very good reason for their being necessary.

On haemodialysis catheters, we have used the technique, and we have identified one unequivocal endarteritis due to a haemodialysis shunt. I have no personal experience of any further data on quantifying infections in haemodialysis catheters.

4 EPIDEMIOLOGY

Professor I. PHILLIPS (London): I would like to take up Dr Dixon's points on the problems of associating the clinical state of a patient with an infusion. Perhaps there are particular problems in the context of low-level contamination.

* See Chapter 7, reference 101

Firstly, many of the patients are not fit healthy people who come in for elective surgery, but people who have had, say, complex operations on the heart valves. These patients have many reasons for being ill. I know of one patient at least who eventually died of a fulminating endocarditis who did not even have a blood culture for twelve days after the operation, although he was clearly ill. The attitude was that all patients got fevers after cardiac surgery and there were other more pressing problems to think about.

Secondly, there may be a tremendous delay. My own hospital has one patient on record who presented about six months after being infused. How is that patient's clinical problem associated with a contaminated infusion?

Finally, sometimes the situation is not as clean as Dr Dixon suggested. In our own outbreak, we were lost in a morass of patients who also had urinary tract infections with the same organism, which, had we recognized the clue, would have led us to the right answer, but which in fact confused us for a time.

Dr DIXON (Boston, Mass.): I certainly agree that epidemiologic evaluations are not always as clean as I have made them seem. They are always cleaner in retrospect.

We had a similar situation with our albumin outbreak; it occurred in a shock trauma unit where all the patients were extremely ill. All of the patients had multiple lines in, and most of the patients had other infections. We were fortunate that two things happened. Firstly, a very astute houseman recognized a unique situation in one patient. The patient had come in with fulminating ulcerative colitis, had to have a colectomy and was recuperating marvellously well. The day before discharge the houseman noticed that the patient's albumin was a little low, and thought that an infusion of albumin might serve as a tonic before discharge. He plugged in the infusion. The patient had a rigor almost immediately, and the houseman having heard about infusion-related bacteraemia wrote down the lot number of the product, cultured it and cultured the blood. It was like money from home, for it implicated a specific batch of albumin; it would have been more difficult but for that. Unfortunately, the episode was not reported to the infection control personnel!

Secondly, how do we really get at the problems of low-frequency contamination and of infection with a common pathogen? One method is to look at aggregate data. Despite the statistical problems of putting dissimilar hospitals together, our studies have shown that surveillance data from a large group of hospitals can be combined to provide quite useful information.

The people who come in much later are a real problem. That is reflected by an outbreak of hepatitis-B disease that was also associated with albumin. The albumin is pasteurised to 60 °C for 10 hours, which supposedly kills hepatitis virus, but one lot of a product was grossly contaminated. Patients came back with typical long-incubation hepatitis. A superb hospital epidemiologist noticed the cluster, and went back to do his shoe-leather epidemiology. Interestingly, since albumin is a biological fluid, the hospital dealt with it in the same way as they did blood; they recorded lot numbers for every patient receiving the product. These numbers solved the hepatitis outbreak.

The substance of this is that for low-frequency events, or for late complications, finding a solution is perhaps 90% luck and 10% good epidemiology. Perhaps good surveillance data will decrease the importance of luck.

Thirdly, background infections. I grant that this is a further problem. It has confused us. Bacteraemias are usually brought to our attention in some dramatic fashion. We always go in with a bias that we must rule out a common source, and approach the problem epidemiologically.

Dr MAKI: On the example quoted by Professor Phillips of urinary tract infections, was it possible in retrospect to identify some common irrigating solution, or something else common to infected patients?

Professor PHILLIPS: In addition to the intravenous fluid, the irrigation fluid was also contaminated, and some of the patients had been attacked from both ends.

Dr MAKI: One thing that Dr Dixon and I have both learnt as part of our experience in the Epidemic Intelligence Service is that a vigorous epidemiological approach to a hospital's problems with a certain type of nosocomial infection is most important, including the use of carefully selected controls when looking at the data. Given, say, many cases of one type of urinary tract infection, one would choose a control group, perhaps patients on the same ward as the patients with infection, or perhaps patients that are age—or sex—matched, or perhaps patients that are matched by having similar kinds of surgery. One would then examine in both cases and controls the entirety of possible related host and therapeutic factors.

I think that one of the most elegant examples of this approach to a nosocomical problem is to be found in a paper on a *Salmonella choleraesuis* outbreak at the National Institutes of Health (Rhame, F. S., Root, R. K., MacLowry, J. D., Dadisman, T. A., and Bennett, J. V. (1973). Salmonella septicaemia from platelet transfusions. *Ann. Int. Med.*, **78**, 633). It was an exceedingly difficult outbreak to crack in that the infections were very infrequent (seven cases over a 6-month period) and widely-spread geographically in a large institute. The analysis went so far as to include factors such as the religion of the patient, but, most important, in both cases and selected controls, eventually pointed to platelet transfusions which had been given in much higher frequency to the infected patients. Even though they cultured hundreds of packs of platelet transfusions with negative results the analysis subsequently showed that a single platelet donor had provided platelets in every case. It turned out that this individual had an asymptomatic case of *Salmonella choleraesuis* osteomylitis with a very low level intermittent bacteraemia. Total volume culturing was necessary to confirm contamination of platelet packs prepared from the donor's blood. The fact that all of the recipients were so immunocompromised permitted occasional sepicaemia to occur, despite the very low level contamination. The epidemiological method—and this primarily —provided the solution to this very complex epidemic problem.

5 PREVENTIVE MEASURES

Mr MYERS: Dr Maki emphasized the dangers of infections from quite a number of points in the giving-set and in the handling of the giving-sets, but when terminal microbial filters were suggested, he felt that the case for them was not proven. Surely the tests that have been carried out on in-line terminal filters have shown that they stop bacteria and particles.

Dr MAKI: I agree that they stop bacteria, but I do not think that the problems have yet been sufficiently worked out. They tend to stop up, and then personnel manipulate the infusions more frequently, and there may be a parodoxically increased risk of infusion-related infection which defeats one of the purposes of the membrane filter, preventing infection.

Membrane filters make a lot of sense in that we know that they stop most bacteria, but they need to be proven effective clinically by controlled trials.

6 TREATMENT

Mr MYERS: Does Dr Jenkins think that intravenous injections of low molecular weight Dextran are of use in these cases?

Dr JENKINS: They are much better than straightforward crystalline solutions. We have very little experience of their use, and we usually use plasma protein in that situation.

Professor PHILLIPS: Does appropriate antibacterial chemotherapy make any difference to the prognosis of patients with the shock syndrome?

Dr DIXON: Obviously it has not been subjected to clinical trials. Our strong clinical impression is that patients having continued infusions through contaminated lines apparently do not do better until the lines are changed, even if they receive appropriate antibotics.

Index

177